EATER'S GUIDE

Candy Cumming, M.S., R.D., is a nutrition consultant to several health-promotion groups. She lectures extensively to community, professional, and corporate groups.

Vicky Newman, M.S., R.D., is a nutritionist and research associate at the University of California Medical Center, San Diego.

Both are charter faculty members of the Sun Valley Health Institute, Idaho, one of the first preventive-medicine programs in the country.

Eater's Guide

Nutrition Basics for Busy People

Candy Cumming
Vicky Newman

A SPECTRUM BOOK

Prentice-Hall, Inc.,
Englewood Cliffs, New Jersey 07632

Library of Congress Cataloging in Publication Data

CUMMING, CANDY.
   Eater's guide.

   (A Spectrum Book)
   Bibliography: p.
   Includes index.
   1. Nutrition.   2. Nutritionally induced diseases—
Prevention.   3. Cookery.   I. Newman, Vicky.   II. Ti-
tle.
QP141.C79   641.5'637   81-232
ISBN 0-13-223057-7   AACR2
ISBN 0-13-223040-2 (pbk.)

This Spectrum Book can be made available to businesses
and organizations at a special discount when ordered
in large quantities. For more information, contact:

     Prentice-Hall, Inc.
     General Book Marketing
     Special Sales Division
     Englewood Cliffs, New Jersey 07632

10 9 8 7 6 5 4 3 2 1

Editorial/production supervision
and interior design by Eric Newman
Cover design by Honi Werner
Manufacturing buyer: Cathie Lenard

Prentice-Hall International, Inc., *London*

Prentice-Hall of Australia Pty. Limited, *Sydney*

Prentice-Hall of Canada, Ltd., *Toronto*

Prentice-Hall of India Private Limited, *New Delhi*

Prentice-Hall of Japan, Inc., *Tokyo*

Prentice-Hall of Southeast Asia Pte. Ltd., *Singapore*

Whitehall Books Limited, *Wellington, New Zealand*

To Vicky's husband, Michael, who kept us well nourished while we wrote this book.

Contents

Preface

If you eat, you need this book. This is especially true if you are a busy person who has some doubts about the way you eat, but little time to learn how to improve your eating style. This book is your source of fast nutrition in a fast-food world.

We've broken down the contents into nineteen brief chapters so that you can bite into one whenever you have five or ten minutes to spare. Or, take an hour or two to digest the whole thing!

You'll find practical suggestions outlining ways to select more natural and healthful foods. We've included some cartoons and humor to tickle your funny bone along the way. And last, but not least, there are many recipes so that you can begin to enjoy this nutrition message right away.

Acknowledgments

This book would not exist if it weren't for some very special people: Jap and May Hammond, Brian Haggerty, and Joan Gussow.

We'd like to thank the Hammonds, two nutrition-conscious people who are really the grandparents of our brainchild, *Eater's Guide*. In 1974, at the age of 74, Jap started his second career by founding the Sun Valley Health Institute (SVHI), one of the first comprehensive health-promotion programs in the country. Since then, Jap and May have inspired thousands of people to choose healthier lifestyles. SVHI provided us with our first opportunity to deliver the nutritional bottom line to Institute participants. It was through our work there that *Eater's Guide* was born.

We also want to give a huge thank you to Brian Haggerty, who taught us the facts of life about publication. Brian was always there with support and helpful advice during the time we sought a publisher. It is impossible to see this book go into print without acknowledging Joan Gussow, Ed.D., our friend and mentor. Joan continues to inspire us to speak out on nutrition issues. As nutritionists we are grateful for her sensitive awareness of the delicate balance of the earth's ecology and the effect of that balance on human life.

EATER'S GUIDE

1
Get Smart

We cannot live without food. It's that simple. But the art of nourishing our bodies has become complicated because food is not simple anymore. Technology has provided us with a plethora of food products that the media woo us to buy. It has become increasingly difficult to sort out the junk from food.

What should we eat? A moderate amount of a wide variety of food is ideal—enough to keep us going, not enough to make us fat. There are no wonder foods. The wonder is that fresh, underprocessed foods possess the nutrients our bodies need to perform their best. Our physical and mental well-being depend a lot on what we eat.

The fifty-odd nutrients that food provides enable our bodies to fuel up and fix up. Just being alive requires "fuelers" for energy; and, as our activity increases, so do our energy needs. Replacement materials ("builders") are also constantly required to replenish the old cells that our bodies slough off each day. "Regulators" are needed to keep all our internal systems functioning smoothly.

Any food worth its oats should provide fuelers and fixers (builders and regulators). The problem with empty calorie (junk) foods is that they contain too much fuel and too little of everything else. Unfortunately, these energy-rich, nutrient-poor foods have become an increasingly greater part of our diet. Refined and processed foods are taking the place of whole grains, fruits, and vegetables.

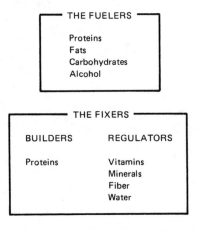

THE FUELERS

Proteins
Fats
Carbohydrates
Alcohol

THE FIXERS

BUILDERS   REGULATORS

Proteins   Vitamins
                  Minerals
                  Fiber
                  Water

These changes in our diet have created nutritional imbalances which increase our vulnerability to several chronic conditions including obesity, heart disease, diabetes, high blood pressure, cancer, dental decay and gum disease, and diverticular disease. Some of these diseases are life-threatening; others are uncomfortable and sap us of our vitality, making us feel older than our years.

Because nutrition plays an important role in the normal functioning of our body's metabolic systems, eating right can improve your general health and help protect you from chronic diseases. The *Dietary Guidelines for Americans* provides information to help us choose a healthier diet. The guidelines in this booklet advise one to

1. Eat a variety of foods.
2. Maintain ideal weight.
3. Avoid too much fat, saturated fat, and cholesterol.
4. Eat foods with adequate starch and fiber.
5. Avoid too much sugar.
6. Avoid too much sodium.
7. (If you drink alcohol) drink only in moderation.

The practicalities of these recommendations will be explained on the pages that follow.

2

How Do You Do?

How healthy is your eating style? To find out, fill in the IQ (Ingestion Questionnaire). Should you discover that you need to modify your nutrition style, fear not! That's what this book is all about.

TABLE 2-1. **Ingestion questionnaire.**

	YOU'RE PRETTY SMART	YOU COULD BE SMARTER
PROTEIN FOODS Part 1: Hidden Fat	___When you eat meat, you select the leanest cuts, like filet mignon, round, sirloin, and veal.	___What's your beef? Is it usually steak, chops, ribs, or hamburger.

	YOU'RE PRETTY SMART	YOU COULD BE SMARTER
PROTEIN FOODS Part 1: Hidden Fat (cont'd.)	____You frequently use poultry, fish, shellfish, tofu (soy bean curd), part- skim cheeses, and legumes (dried peas and beans).	____You frequently eat cold cuts, hot dogs, and full-fat cheeses like jack and cheddar.
		____Quiche Lorraine is your token "natural" food.
	____You use nonfat or lowfat milk as a beverage and in cooking most of the time.	____You regularly use whole milk, cream, and half-and-half as a beverage and in cooking.
	____You infrequently use whole milk and cream.	YOU'RE GETTING LOTS OF FAT: CHECK CHAPTERS 7 and 8 FOR THE FAT FACTS OF LIFE.
Part 2: Cholesterol	____You seldom eat more than 6 oz. (cooked weight) of meat daily.	____You like big portions of meat, so you usually eat more than 8 oz. of it each day.
	____When you eat eggs, you have them poached or cooked with a minimal amount of fat.	____You like your eggs smothered with fat, so you usually eat omelettes or fried or scrambled eggs.
		TO UNSCRAMBLE THE CONFUSION ABOUT CHOLESTEROL, CHECK CHAPTER 10.

TABLE 2-1 (cont'd.).

	YOU'RE PRETTY SMART	YOU COULD BE SMARTER
FAT FOODS	___You use all spreads (butter, margarine, mayonnaise) and salad dressings sparingly.	___You have a heavy hand with spreads, salad dressings, dips, sour cream, oils.
	___You seldom eat fried or fast foods.	___You eat a lot of fried or fast food.
		___Into the energy crunch? You frequently use nuts and seeds as a snack.
		YOU MIGHT BE GETTING MORE FAT THAN YOU THINK! CHECK CHAPTER 7 AGAIN.
	___You use milk to lighten coffee or tea.	___You usually use a nondairy creamer as a lightener.
	___You use crackers and cereals that do not contain added fats.	___You frequently eat granola and granola bars.
		___You use diet meal replacements like Figurines.
		___You eat a lot of packaged cakes, cookies, and chips.
		___You use a solid vegetable shortening for cooking.
		___You frequently use convenience foods and mixes.
		READ CHAPTER 9 TO SEE IF YOU HAVE BEEN FOOLING AROUND WITH MOTHER NATURE.

	YOU'RE PRETTY SMART	YOU COULD BE SMARTER
CARBO-HYDRATES: Part 1: Fiber Foods	___You include at least one of the following daily: citrus fruits, cantaloupe, strawberries, deep green leafy vegetables, cauliflower, broccoli, cabbage, brussel sprouts, peppers (green or chili), tomatoes.	___Usually, you eat less than one serving daily of the foods listed in the opposite column.
	___Your salads are full of a variety of vegetables including deep greens like romaine and spinach.	___You eat salads that consist mostly of head lettuce.
	___You include deep green or yellow vegetables in your daily diet.	___You skimp on vegetables, seldom eat those that are deep green or yellow.
	___You eat at least four servings a day of fruits and vegetables.	___You usually have less than 4 servings a day of fruits and vegetables.
		BUILD YOUR IMMUNITY AGAINST INFECTIONS AND DISEASES, LIKE CANCER. GO BACK TO "THE SOURCE," CHAPTER 17, FOR FOODS HIGH IN VITAMIN C.
	___You use whole fruits often.	___You drink juices instead of eating whole fruits.

TABLE 2-1 (cont'd.).

	YOU'RE PRETTY SMART	YOU COULD BE SMARTER
CARBO-HYDRATES: Part 1: Fiber Foods (cont'd.)	____Most of your starches are whole grains.	____You generally eat white breads, refined cereals, and white rice. ____You tend to avoid all starches because "they're fattening." YOU'RE LOSING FIBER! HOW WILL YOU EVER MAKE A FLUFFY? WHAT'S A FLUFFY? SEE CHAPTER 5. WHILE YOU'RE AT IT, READ CHAPTERS 3 & 4, TOO.
Part 2: Sweet Foods	____You seldom eat desserts and candies. ____You munch on fruits or vegetables for desserts and snacks. ____You make an effort to use less sugar when preparing a dessert item. ____You use unsweetened cereals. ____You drink fruit juice without added sugar.	____You usually have one or more of the following daily: donuts, cake, sweet rolls, cookies, pie, jello, fruited yogurt or frozen yogurt, ice cream, sherbet, ice milk, candy, chocolate milk, hot chocolate, shakes, fruit canned in heavy syrup. ____You use presweetened cereals (including "natural," granola-type cereals.) ____You drink soft drinks, Tang, and other fruit-flavored drinks.

	YOU'RE PRETTY SMART	YOU COULD BE SMARTER
Part 2: Sweet Foods (cont'd.)	____You use sugar, honey, syrup, and jams sparingly.	____You use liberal amounts of all sweeteners, including sugar, honey, and jam.
	____You avoid artificial sweeteners and products that contain them.	____You use artificial sweeteners, diet pop, etc.
		____You've been sweet talked into using fructose. YOU MIGHT BE SWEETER THAN YOU THINK. SEE CHAPTER 6.
SALTY FOODS	____You use fresh meats and legumes.	____You use processed foods like hot dogs, cold cuts, sausages, processed cheeses, textured soy products (Morning-star Farms, for example)
	____You use fresh vegetables or those that have been frozen with little or no salt.	____You use canned vegetables and those frozen with salt, sauces, and monosodium glutamate.
	____You use very little salt in cooking.	____You season generously with salt, MSG (Accent), soy sauce, seasoned salts, and sea salt.
	____You seldom use the salt shaker at the table.	____You usually salt foods after they have been prepared.

9

TABLE 2-1 (cont'd.).

	YOU'RE PRETTY SMART	YOU COULD BE SMARTER
SALTY FOODS (cont'd)	___You season with herbs, spices, wine, garlic, and onion.	___You use a lot of packaged sauces, canned soups, and bouillon cubes. ___You frequently use salted chips, nuts, crackers, and pretzels. ___You often rely on convenience foods like TV dinners and fast foods. OOPS! PERHAPS YOU NEED TO GET INTO A SALT AGREEMENT. SALT TALKS BEGIN IN CHAPTER 11.
BEVERAGES	___You drink water to quench thirst. ___You rarely drink more than 2 cups of coffee or tea daily.	___You seldom drink water. ___You drink plenty of coffee, tea, cola beverages, Dr Pepper, Mountain Dew, or hot chocolate. YOU'VE GOT SOME NERVE! CHECK WHAT'S BREWING, CHAPTER 12.
	___You average one alcoholic drink or less a day.	___You average more than one drink per day. FOR A POLLUTION SOLUTION OR SOME CHEER, READ CHAPTER 13.

	YOU'RE PRETTY SMART	YOU COULD BE SMARTER
WEIGHT CONTROL	___You stay within an ideal weight range for your height and build.	___You usually weigh more than your ideal body weight.
	___You seldom overeat.	___You frequently overeat.
	___You eat slowly.	___You eat very rapidly.
	___You seldom eat while otherwise occupied.	___You often eat while engaged in other activities like reading, watching TV, cooking, and talking on the phone.
	___When you eat, you are usually hungry.	___You often eat when you are not hungry.
	___You seldom use food for reasons other than the satisfaction of hunger.	___You frequently use food when upset, sad, depressed, anxious, happy, procrastinating, etc.
	___You eat regularly and plan for meals and snacks.	___You frequently raid the refrigerator.
	___You consider physical activity to be an important part of weight control, so you exercise regularly.	___You seldom exercise. LEARN HOW TO FIGHT FAT. BOLT TO A "LIGHTENING" SUBJECT. SEE CHAPTER 14.
	___You eat a wide variety of nutritious foods, and a minimum of "goodies."	___You often follow "crash" diets.
		___You follow a high protein diet to lose weight.

TABLE 2-1 (cont'd.).

	YOU'RE PRETTY SMART	YOU COULD BE SMARTER
WEIGHT CONTROL (cont'd)		CONTROLLING WEIGHT WITH GROUPS MAY HELP YOU OUT. LEARN HOW IN CHAPTER 15. YOU MIGHT NEED A SUPPLEMENT. CHECK CHAPTER 18.
	___You indulge yourself from time to time with a rich food without feeling guilty.	___You feel guilty when breaking a diet.
	___You set realistic weight loss goals (1 to 2 lb weight loss weekly.)	___You set unrealistic weight loss goals.
	___You encourage yourself toward successful management of your weight.	___You discourage yourself with a lot of negative talk when you mismanage your weight.
		EXPAND YOUR MIND. SHRINK YOUR BODY. CHAPTER 14 IS FOR YOU.

3

Beef Up Your Diet with Beans

Just about everyone knows that protein is important for health. Unfortunately, many people think that the more protein they get, the healthier they become. This misconception has led most of us to believe that protein foods are truly wonder foods, and that our diets should be full of protein—especially from meat.

Actually, getting enough protein is not the problem. The problem is that we get too much. Blessed with plentiful food, Americans have been eating excess protein for years. Although we used to get a lot of our protein from starchy foods like grains, potatoes, vegetables, and beans, today we have become hooked on meat—especially big juicy steaks, chops, and burgers.

Admittedly, meat is a good source of protein. It is also full of fat. Cutting down on meat is a good idea because every ounce provides one and a half times more calories from fat than from protein. So if your diet consists mostly of meats, you are really on a high-fat as well as a high-protein diet!

A rediscovery of nutritional truths spotlights the fact that carbohydrates can be "good guys" after all. So try replacing some of your meat with *unrefined* carbohydrate foods such as grains, potatoes, vegetables, and beans. This will decrease your intake of fat and cholesterol. The unrefined carbohydrates will also add color and crunch, and important vitamins, minerals and fiber to your diet.

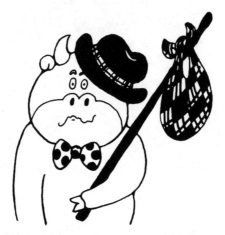

Eating a lot of beef is a bum steer!

For those of us brought up on meat, it seems impossible that life could be sustained without it. Yet some vegetarian groups appear to be healthier than the average American. Research on vegetarians who eat eggs and milk products indicates that, in comparison with average Americans, vegetarians have

1. Lower serum cholesterol and lower serum triglycerides.
2. One-third the risk of developing fatal heart disease.
3. Less high blood pressure.

4. A lower incidence of many cancers including breast, colon, and rectum.
5. Less osteoporosis or softening of the bones.
6. Fewer bowel problems, like diverticular disease.

We realize that you're not going to rush out and become a vegetarian overnight because of this information. But we would like you to consider adding more vegetarian meals to your diet, both for variety and for your health.

To produce a nourishing vegetarian meal, you need to know a little about protein. There is a fundamental difference between animal and vegetable protein. An animal protein generally contains all the amino acids (protein building blocks) necessary to produce and maintain body tissue. A vegetable protein, on the other hand, is usually low in one or more of these amino acid building blocks. Consequently, a vegetable protein needs to be mixed with another protein, *either* animal or vegetable, that will supply the insufficient amino acid. This process is known as complementary protein combination. (See Figure 3-1 for more information.)

You may notice that a number of vegetarian dishes are made with cheddar or another high-fat cheese. Don't be alarmed. Usually the recipes call for one cup (four ounces) of grated cheese to serve four people. This means that each portion is still quite low in saturated fat content, especially if you compare it with the typical (six-ounce) serving of meat.

A vegetarian diet only presents problems when all animal products are eliminated. On such strict regimes, pregnant and breastfeeding women, as well as young children, may have difficulty obtaining adequate amounts of protein, vitamin B-12, calcium, iron, and zinc. In fact, a supplement of vitamin B-12 is recommended if no milk products or eggs are eaten, because this vitamin is present almost exclusively in foods of animal origin.

Learning about the combinations that yield high-quality protein is an adventure into a new world of intriguing tastes, textures, and colors. In addition, eating more vegetable protein adds extra vitamins,

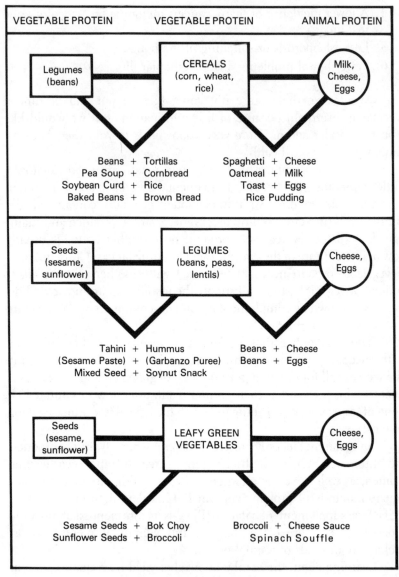

FIGURE 3-1. **Complementary protein combination.**

minerals, and fiber to your daily fare. Cutting down on the amount of animal foods that you eat also helps to reduce the fat and cholesterol content of your meals.

For more information on vegetarian diets, read *Laurel's Kitchen* and the *Nutrition Survival Kit* (see the Suggested Reading List in Appendix C). You may also wish to try some of the vegetarian recipes included in this book for some delightful dining (see Chapter 20).

Ban the Bread?

Many of us shy away from carbohydrates. We think that they are fattening, and we munch on more meat instead. Yet breads, potatoes, and legumes (beans, peas, and lentils) were the mainstay of our ancestors' diets. Don't you think it strange that we, conscious of cutting carbohydrate calories, are fatter than they were? Replacing starchy foods with meat has actually made our diets richer in fat. Ounce for ounce, fats have twice the calories of carbohydrates. Whoever said "ban the bread" has misled a lot of us!

Whole grains, fresh potatoes, vegetables, and legumes provide our bodies with valuable nutrients including protein, B-vitamins, trace minerals like iron, and fiber. A large portion of these nutrients is removed during processing. The enrichment program followed in some states requires that at least thiamin, riboflavin, niacin, and iron be

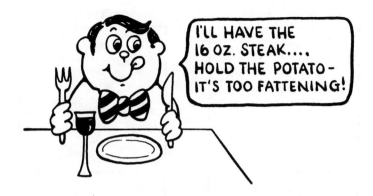

I'LL HAVE THE 16 OZ. STEAK.... HOLD THE POTATO—IT'S TOO FATTENING!

added back to refined grain products like flour and rice. Unfortunately, several other key nutrients (including vitamin B-6, folic acid, pantothenic acid, vitamin E, magnesium, zinc, and selenium) that are seriously depleted by the refining process are not added back. Moreover, the form of iron added to most enriched products is poorly absorbed. Therefore, though enriched products are better than those not enriched, they certainly are not as nourishing as whole grains.

Sugar is so highly refined that it retains essentially none of the vitamins, minerals, or fiber found in the beets, corn, or cane from which it is derived. Therefore, it is best to avoid sugars, flours, grains, and potatoes that have been refined. Unfortunately, these are the carbohydrates that we are eating in increasingly larger amounts today.

Switching to more unrefined fruits, vegetables, grains, and legumes can actually help control obesity by decreasing overconsumption and absorption of calories. These foods also contain lots of plant fiber, which has recently been shown to be beneficial in the prevention and treatment of diabetes, heart disease, certain types of cancer, and a variety of gastrointestinal problems.

To help us avoid the pain and discomfort of these diseases, the *Dietary Guidelines for Americans* recommends that we eat more wholesome carbohydrate foods (see Figure 4-1). Suggestions for doing this follow, and can also be found in Chapters 5 and 6.

1. Eat more legumes (beans, peas, lentils), potatoes, and other vegetables.

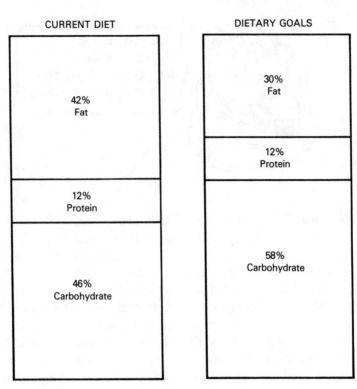

FIGURE 4-1. **Current diet and dietary goals.**

2. Eat whole-grain breads and cereals daily.
   - Be sure the label says *whole, sprouted,* or *malted* grain as the first ingredient.
   - Don't be fooled by the words *wheat flour;* they mean white flour.
   - If you don't like whole-wheat bread, use old-fashioned oatmeal or Shredded Wheat in the morning.
3. Consume whole fresh fruits instead of fruit juices or fruit-flavored drinks.
4. Try to have a raw fruit or vegetable with each meal, preferably one rich in vitamin C or folic acid (see Chapter 17).

5. Try to replace six teaspoons of your current fat intake with the equivalent calories in all of the following:
   - 2 slices whole-wheat bread
   - 1 small potato
   - 1 cup dark green leafy vegetable
   - 1 small orange

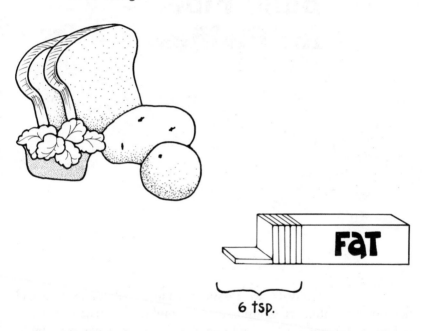

6 tsp.

That's a lot of color, crunch, and food volume for an equivalent number of calories. Wouldn't you feel really satisfied with all that extra food?

You see, there's really no reason to ban good bread after all!

5

The Incredible Bulk: Fiber for Fluffies

Every day we are subjected to TV ads for laxatives and hemorrhoid ointments. Considering the number of such commercials, it appears that constipation and hemorrhoids are very common problems.

Insufficient intake of fiber-rich foods interferes with the healthy functioning of your intestinal tract. Aside from difficulties with constipation and hemorrhoids, some serious illnesses like gallbladder disease, diverticulosis, and cancer of the colon and rectum appear to be more common among people whose diets are low in plant fiber.

Without the regular stimulation provided by adequate fiber, the rhythmic contractions of your intestines are less frequent. Thus the intestinal muscles become weakened and the stool becomes hard, because the longer it sits in the large intestine, the more water is resorbed from it.

It is currently believed that the intestinal pouches of diverticulosis result when the pressure caused by straining at stool is coupled with weakened intestinal muscles. When these pouches become inflamed, the condition is known as *diverticulitis*. A diet high in plant fiber has recently been shown to be effective in the treatment of diverticulosis.

Current medical literature also implicates our low-fiber, high-fat, and high-animal-protein diet as a cause of cancer of the colon (large intestine) and rectum. Though the reasons are not clear, populations eating more fiber (from real food, not from purified wood pulp) and less fat and protein (especially less from animal sources), seem to develop less of these types of cancer.

The recent advertising of new high-fiber cereals has sparked a lot of public interest. A frequent question is: "How do I know I am getting enough fiber?" To answer this question, use your own built-in feedback mechanism—your stool. Large, "fluffy" soft stools are the result of a high-fiber diet. Small, hard stools result from a diet low in fiber. Because diseases of the intestine are serious and painful, it is important to remember what to eat to produce "fluffies."

Unprocessed bran is one type of fiber that comes from the coating of the wheat kernel. Adding bran to your cereals, meat loaf, hamburgers, salads, and breads is one way to increase the fiber content of your diet. Generally speaking, however, *a diet that is plentiful in a variety of whole grains, fruits, vegetables, and legumes is a better bet.* The different types of fiber that these foods contain perform different functions in the body. Bran, for example, is helpful in relieving constipation and in the treatment of diverticular disease. But other types of fiber, particularly those found in oats, citrus, and legumes appear to be more effective in lowering serum cholesterol and in protecting from gallbladder disease.

During periods when you cannot eat a variety of fiber-rich foods to maintain regularity, you can try adding two to four tablespoons of bran to your daily diet. Start with one tablespoon of bran and gradually increase until you get the results you want. Remember to increase liquids and brisk exercise at the same time, as these also help to insure regularity.

Foods high in fiber are also "bulky." They take up a lot of room in your stomach, thus satisfying your hunger with fewer calories. Refined foods, on the other hand, slide down quite easily. Consider chocolate cake à la mode—600 calories down the hatch in a few melt-in-your-mouth moments. Trading that snack in for its caloric equivalent in fruit would mean eating fifteen pieces. Imagine munching on all that! Thus, a diet high in fiber-rich foods can also help to control your weight.

6
Sweet Teeth Bite, Too

Our sweet tooth bites a huge chunk out of our daily diet, making sugar and corn sweeteners account for almost one-fifth of the calories we eat. That averages out to about *twelve tablespoons* of sugar daily! Of course, we don't sprinkle that much sugar onto our food. The majority of it comes already added to the convenience foods, desserts, and soft drinks that we gobble up and guzzle down. In fact, the largest increase in the use of refined sugar has been in beverages such as soft drinks, the consumption of which has more than doubled in the past fifteen years. Today the average American drinks about 330 twelve-ounce cans of soda each year.

To become more aware of the hidden sugar in the foods you eat, see Table 6-1. Each "S" represents one tablespoon of sugar.

Some breakfast cereals contain so much sugar that it would prob-

TABLE 6-1. **Hidden sugar.**

1 slice cake, iced	SSSS
12-oz. can of soda	SSS
1 cup jello	SSS
1 slice fruit pie	SSS
1 slice custard cream pie	SS
1 cup flavored yogurt	SS
1/2 cup sherbet	SS
1 glazed donut	SS
1 plain donut	S
1/2 cup ice cream	S
1 ice cream cone	S
2 small cookies	S
1/2 cup pudding	S
1/2 cup canned fruit	S
1/2 cup sweetened cereal	S
1 candy bar	S

ably be more accurate to call them candy. See Table 6-2 for the sugar content of cereals.

Your best bet is to buy whole-grain cereals with *no* added sugar. It is also a good idea to avoid those cereals fortified with vitamin D, as this vitamin has already been added to most milk and large amounts are not healthy.

Don't let sugar's other names fool you. Sugar is often disguised on a label as corn syrup, fructose, dextrose, or glucose. Raw, brown, and turbinado are also just other names for sugar. Incidentally, honey and fructose are no sweet bargain, in spite of current claims. They're concentrated sweeteners just like all the others. Avoid buying foods listing any of these sweeteners as one of the first three ingredients.

TABLE 6-2. **Here's the sugar* in your morning munchy.**

0 TO 5% SUGAR	
Shredded Wheat	Branola
Oatmeal	Roman Meal
Whole Wheat Cereal	Wheatena
Wheat Hearts	Cream of Wheat

0 TO 5% SUGAR

Cheerios	Alpen
Puffed Rice	Post Toasties
Uncle Sam Cereal	Product 19
Wheat Chex	Corn Total
Grape Nut Flakes	Special K
Puffed Wheat	Wheaties

6 TO 20% SUGAR

Corn Flakes	Heartland (with raisins)
Grape Nuts	Buck Wheat
Crispy Rice	Life
Corn Chex	Granola Cereals
Total	Sugar Frosted Corn Flakes
Rice Chex	40% Bran Flakes
Crisp Rice	Team
Raisin Bran	Granola
Concentrate	100% Bran Cereal
Rice Crispies	All Bran

21 TO 40% SUGAR

Fortified Oat Flakes	Frosted Mini Wheats
Heartland	Sugar Pops
Super Sugar Chex	Alpha Bits
Sugar Frosted Flakes	Sir Grapefellow
Bran Buds	Super Sugar Crisp
Sugar Sparkled Corn Flakes	

41 TO 50% SUGAR

Cocoa Puffs	Vanilly Crunch
Cap'n Crunch	Baron Von Redberry
Crunch Berries	Cocoa Krispies
Kaboom	Trix
Frankenberry	Froot Loops
Frosted Flakes	Honeycomb
Count Chocula	Pink Panther
Orange Quangaroos	Cinnamon Crunch
Quisp	Lucky Charms
Boo Berry	

MORE THAN 50% SUGAR

Cocoa Pebbles	King Vitaman
Apple Jacks	Sugar Smacks
Fruity Pebbles	Super Orange Crisp

*Sugar percent by weight based on Shannon (1974).

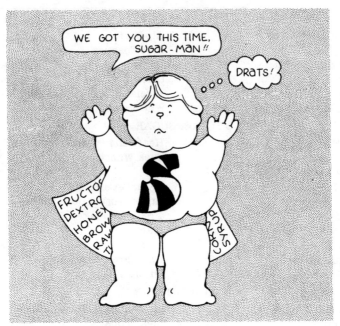

Sugar Man is often disguised
as glucose, fructose,
dextrose, corn syrup, corn
syrup solids, raw sugar,
brown sugar, turbinado,
and—even—your honey!

You may now be wondering whether to replace sugar with saccharin. We recommend that you don't because of saccharin's questionable safety. It's better to learn to decrease your sugar habit slowly than to replace a real sweet with a fake one. You'll be surprised at the subtle, wonderful taste of real food.

Remember, when you add the sugar, you have control. In recipes calling for sugar, reduce the amount you add by a third to a half. Start to think of sugar as a seasoning, not as the primary ingredient in a recipe. For example, a bit of sugar added to an oil and vinegar dressing helps to cut the tartness of the vinegar. This is better than diluting the vinegar with large amounts of high-calorie oil.

It's not difficult to cut down on the sugar you consume. Just follow these few guidelines.

1. At snack time, munch on fruits and raw vegetables, whole grains, and lowfat dairy products instead of soft drinks, cakes, candies, and cookies.
2. After meals, substitute fruit or milk desserts for cookies, cakes, and pies.
3. Sweeten cereal with fruit instead of sugar.
4. Avoid adding sugar to coffee and tea.
5. Drink water instead of sweetened beverages during and between meals.
6. Try replacing soda with a mixture of half soda water and half fruit juice.

Next time you want to reach for a sweet, remember what happens when you eat too much sugar.

She was the picture of refinement!

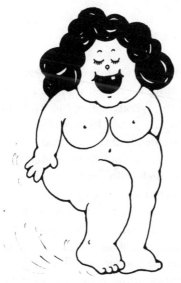

7
Rats!
Those Fats!

Americans love fatty foods—all that butter, oil, margarine, and salad dressing we spread on bread, pour over greens, and smear on top of crackers. We are eating more fats now than ever before and it is not doing us any good. In fact, the increased consumption of all kinds of fats (saturated and unsaturated) is believed to contribute to heart disease. There is also increasing evidence correlating high-fat, high-protein, low-fiber diets with certain forms of cancer—particularly cancer of the breast, uterus, prostate, colon, and rectum. Just a few alterations in your current dietary habits could greatly reduce your risk of these two diseases. But first, you need to know more about fat.

There are several forms of fats. Visible fats include all the obvious sources like butter, cream, margarine, oil, mayonnaise, salad dressings, and the strip of fat surrounding meat. Invisible fats are the insidious ones hidden in meat, milk, nuts, cold cuts, and cheese. And finally, there are the fats we would rather not admit to—those found in our favorite "goodies"—ice cream, cookies, cakes, donuts, candies, pastries, and crackers. Even "natural" breakfast cereals like granola contain a considerable amount of fat.

You can actually determine how much fat you usually eat by using the "Fats in Your Life" chart (Table 7-1). Remember, according to the *Dietary Goals for the United States,* only 30 percent of your calories should come from fat.

Figure your approximate daily calories by multiplying your weight by twelve (if you are not very active) or by fifteen (if you are moderately active). For example, if you weigh 150 pounds and are not very active, you require approximately 1800 calories daily to maintain your weight. Once you have figured your daily calories, consult Table 7-1 to see how many grams of fat would equal 30 percent of your daily calories. Then you can determine the amount of fat in your diet and see how close you come to the recommended amount.

TABLE 7-1. **The fats in your life.**

DAILY CALORIES	30% CALORIES = GRAMS FAT
1200	40
1500	50
1800	60
2100	70
2400	80
2700	90
3000	100

	FOOD	SERVING SIZE	FAT (GM)
BREAD	Biscuit	2" diameter	5
PRODUCTS	Corn bread	2" × 2" × 1"	5
	Crackers, buttery (Ritz, Triscuits)	5	5
	Granola	1/4 cup	5
	Muffin, plain	2" diameter	5

TABLE 7-1 (cont'd.).

	FOOD	SERVING SIZE	FAT (GM)
BREAD PRODUCTS (cont'd.)	Pancake or waffle	5" × 1/2" diameter	5
	Potatoes, french-fried	8 (2" × 3 1/2")	10
	Potato or corn chips	15	10
DAIRY PRODUCTS	Cheese, cottage, dry or low-fat	1/2 cup	2
	Cheese, cottage, creamed	1/2 cup	5
	Cheese, mozzarella, ricotta, farmer's, and neufchatel	1 ounce	4
	Cheese, parmesan	3 tablespoons	5
	Cheese, cheddar, jack	1 ounce	8
	Milk and yogurt, low-fat	8 ounces	5
	Milk and yogurt, whole	8 ounces	10
FATS	Avocado	1/8 of 4" diameter	5
	Bacon fat or lard	1 teaspoon	5
	Bacon, crisp	1 strip	5
	Butter	1 teaspoon	4
	Cream, heavy (whipping)	2 tablespoons	10
	Cream, light (half and half)	2 tablespoons	5
	Cream, sour	2 tablespoons	5
	Cream cheese	2 tablespoons	10
	Margarine	1 teaspoon	4
	Mayonnaise	1 teaspoon	4
	Mayonnaise, low-calorie	1 teaspoon	2
	Oil	1 teaspoon	5
	Olives	5 small	5
	Salad dressing, creamy style	1 tablespoon	7
	Salad dressing, oil-vinegar style	1 tablespoon	5
PROTEIN, ANIMAL	Beef, baby, chipped, chuck, flank, tenderloin, round, sirloin, heart	1 ounce	3
	Beef, ground (15% fat), corned beef (canned), rib eye, ground round (commercial)	1 ounce	6

	FOOD	SERVING SIZE	FAT (GM)
PROTEIN, ANIMAL (cont'd.)	Beef, brisket, ground (commercial, more than 20% fat), roasts (rib), steaks (club and rib)	1 ounce	8
	Cold cuts	1 ounce	8
	Egg	1 medium	6
	Fish, any fresh or frozen (except salmon and rainbow trout)	1 ounce	1
	Fish, salmon, rainbow trout, tuna (canned in oil)	1 ounce or 1/4 cup	4
	Fish, clams, crab, lobster, oysters, scallops, shrimp	1 ounce	1
	Fish, sardines, drained	3	3
	Frankfurter	1 standard	10
	Lamb, leg, rib, sirloin, loin (roast/chops), shank, shoulder	1 ounce	3
	Pork, leg, ham, smoked	1 ounce	3
	Pork, tenderloin, shoulder (picnic), Boston Butt, Canadian bacon, boiled ham	1 ounce	6
	Pork, spare ribs, loin, ground, deviled ham	1 ounce	8
	Poultry, chicken, turkey (without skin)	1 ounce	1
	Poultry, chicken, turkey (with skin)	1 ounce	2
	Poultry, capon, duck, goose	1 ounce	8
	Veal, all cuts except breast	1 ounce	3
	Variety meats, liver, kidney, sweetbreads	1 ounce	3
PROTEIN, VEGE- TABLE	Almonds	10 whole	5
	Nuts, others not named	6 small	5
	Pecans	2 large whole	5
	Peanuts, Spanish	20 whole	5
	Peanuts, Virginia	10 whole	5

TABLE 7-1 (cont'd.).

	FOOD	SERVING SIZE	FAT (GM)
PROTEIN, VEGE- TABLE	Peanut butter	1 tablespoon	8
	Seeds	1 tablespoon	5
	Walnuts	4-5 halves	5
SWEETS	Cake, no icing	3″ × 3″ × 2″ piece	8
	Cake, with icing	3″ × 3″ × 2″ piece	18
	Cheesecake	1/9 of 9″ cake	35
	Cookie	1 medium	3
	Ice cream	1/2 cup	10
	Pie, fruit, cream, custard	1/6 of 9″ pie	18
	Pie, pecan	1/6 of 9″ pie	35
	Sherbet	1/2 cup	5

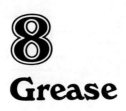

Grease

Polyunsaturated, hydrogenated, saturated, partially hardened. You've probably seen these words on thousands of labels. Do you know what they mean?

The adjective used to describe a fat tells you secrets about its physical form and how it affects your body. It is the amount of hydrogen in the fat molecule that determines its degree of saturation and its hardness. The harder the fat is at room temperature, the more saturated it is. In general, animal fats are harder and more saturated than naturally occurring vegetable fats.

Saturated fats are full of hydrogen, so they are solid or semisolid at room temperature. In excessive amounts, saturated fats have a tendency to raise the body's serum cholesterol level, thus increasing the risk of heart disease. While you have heard that meat and dairy fats

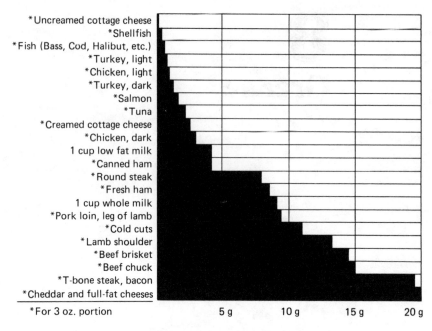

*Uncreamed cottage cheese			
*Shellfish			
*Fish (Bass, Cod, Halibut, etc.)			
*Turkey, light			
*Chicken, light			
*Turkey, dark			
*Salmon			
*Tuna			
*Creamed cottage cheese			
*Chicken, dark			
1 cup low fat milk			
*Canned ham			
*Round steak			
*Fresh ham			
1 cup whole milk			
*Pork loin, leg of lamb			
*Cold cuts			
*Lamb shoulder			
*Beef brisket			
*Beef chuck			
*T-bone steak, bacon			
*Cheddar and full-fat cheeses			

*For 3 oz. portion

5 g   10 g   15 g   20 g

Other sources of saturated fats: coconut and palm oils, cocoa butter, lard, butterfat, hydrogenated oils, household shortening

FIGURE 8-1. **Saturated fat content of foods.**

are saturated, you may be surprised to learn that several vegetable fats are also saturated. These include palm oil, coconut oil, and cocoa butter. If you become a label reader, you will notice the frequency with which these vegetable fats are used in crackers, "natural" cereals, nondairy creamers, and other convenience foods.

You may not have heard of the term *monounsaturated* before, but you're surely familiar with this type of fat. Monounsaturated fats are found in some of your favorite foods—avocados, peanuts, olives, and most nuts (except walnuts which are high in "polys"). Oils derived from these "monos" are liquid at room temperature, but become thick when refrigerated. They neither raise nor lower your serum cholesterol.

Polyunsaturated fats are the ones you hear touted on TV frequently; they have gotten "good press." We are led to believe that using a lot of "polys" will magically cure heart disease. This, however, is a misleading claim. Like other fats, the "polys" should be used sparingly. When you reduce your saturated fat intake as suggested, the "polys" that are in your diet help to lower your serum cholesterol level.

Polyunsaturated fats are found most abundantly in plants. They are liquid at room temperature and remain liquid even when refrigerated. "Polys" are excellent sources of linoleic acid, a nutrient needed for healthy skin and for blood pressure regulation. Highest in polyunsaturates are sunflower, safflower, and corn oils. Soy, sesame, and cottonseed oils are also polyunsaturated, though less so. It is a good idea to keep these oils tightly covered and to store them in a cool, dark place to avoid rancidity.

Remember, your body needs a variety of natural (saturated, monounsaturated, and polyunsaturated) fats daily. But use them all sparingly in an effort to reduce total fat consumption. Here are some suggestions to help you get started.

1. Limit beef, pork, lamb, and cheeses made from whole milk to a combined total of 16 ounces per week.
   - Each ounce of these contains approximately 1 teaspoon of saturated fat.
   - A piece of cooked meat the size of your palm weighs about 3 to 4 ounces.
   - A 1″ cube or 1/4 cup of grated cheese weighs about an ounce.
2. Replace red meat with poultry, fish, and legumes several times a week.
3. When you do eat meat, select the leanest cuts and remove all visible fat and skin before eating (See Group I in Meat Exchanges, Appendix A).
4. Try to avoid luncheon meats, frankfurters, and sausage because they are so high in fat.
5. Skim the fat off broths, soups, and gravies.
6. Bake, broil, or boil meats more often. Try to avoid frying. If you do sauté, use small amounts of oil with, perhaps, a tad of butter for extra flavor.

7. Switch to nonfat or lowfat milk.
   - Whole milk contains the equivalent of 2 teaspoons butter per cup.
   - Lowfat milk contains only about 1 teaspoon of butter per cup.
   - Nonfat milk contains no butter.
   - If you prefer whole milk, you can reduce your intake of fats from other sources to compensate.
8. Try to use cheeses made with part-skim milk rather than those made with whole milk. Recommended cheeses include
   - Cottage, farmer
   - Ricotta, mozzarella
   - Gruyère, Jarlesberg Swiss
   - Sapsago
9. Use only small portions of mashed avocado, fresh butter, margarine (listing liquid oil as the first ingredient), and mayonnaise.
10. Use salad dressings sparingly.
    - One 1/4-cup (the amount contained in most salad-bar ladles) may contain as much as 200 calories of fat.
    - Try diluting cheesy salad dressings and mayonnaise with buttermilk or lowfat yogurt to decrease the fat content.
11. Avoid rich dishes made with butter and cream, and try not to use products made with palm, coconut oil, or cocoa butter.

9

Foolin' Around
with Mother Nature

Can you really fool Mother Nature? The makers of leading brands of margarine tell us that their products are as tasty as butter, only healthier. But the enthusiasm for margarine results more from advertising and its relatively low price than from a close look at the facts.

Margarine is not the same as the oil from which it is made. Several significant changes take place during production which results in hydrogenation, or hardening, of the oil to differing degrees. The more hydrogen that is added, the more saturated and harder the margarine becomes. Simply put, this is how a liquid oil turns into a hard stick of margarine or a "plastic" shortening. Unfortunately, many of the beneficial qualities of the polyunsaturated oil are lost during the

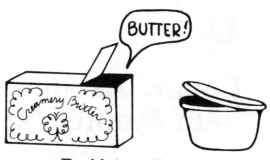

The debate continues...

hydrogenation process. In addition, much of the essential fatty acid, linoleic acid, is destroyed.

Hydrogenation produces a rare type of fat molecule that seldom occurs in nature. Such fats are called "trans" fatty acids. The popularity of processed convenience foods, as well as misleading claims for margarine, has brought about a dramatic increase in the amount of hydrogenated fats and trans fatty acids that we eat. The use of margarine has increased about eightfold and shortening more than twofold since 1909.

Although trans fatty acids can provide energy, recent research indicates that they do not function appropriately in several systems in our body. It appears that trans fats have an adverse effect on the structure and function of our cells, and may even jeopardize our cardiovascular and hormonal systems. It would seem that ol' Ma Nature can't be fooled after all.

If you eat margarine, pick one listing liquid oil as the first ingredient. This shows that there is a higher proportion of polyunsaturated oil to hydrogenated oil. The margarine would, therefore, have fewer of the negative characteristics associated with hydrogenation. The most healthful thing to do, however, is to go easy on all fats and to eat only those fats that have undergone a minimal amount of processing.

Here are a few more suggestions to help you stop fooling around with Mother Nature. After all, the joke may be on you.

1. Steer clear of products containing hydrogenated fats. These include
   - Crackers, cookies, cakes, and granola bars
   - Candy bars
   - Nondairy creamers
   - Diet meal replacements (Figurines, etc.)
   - Most fast foods
2. For your occasional sweet treat, use fresh butter instead of margarine or shortening.
   - When you eat the real thing, the flavor is much more satisfying.
   - But remember, rich desserts are for special occasions and are not meant to be eaten every day.

10

Cracking
the Cholesterol
Controversy

During the past few decades, cholesterol has received a lot of bad press. It has been blamed as the dietary cause of heart disease. Because of its notorious reputation, many people are unaware of the vital role that this fat-like compound plays in the body.

Cholesterol is the raw material from which sex hormones and cortisone are made. A cholesterol-related substance is found beneath the skin's surface, where it is transformed into vitamin D in the presence of sunlight. Bile acids, needed for the digestion of fat, require cholesterol for their production by the liver. Cholesterol is also part of the structure of all the nerves in the body and is a major component of the brain.

Even though cholesterol is vital to normal body functioning, an elevated cholesterol level in the blood is associated with an increased risk of heart disease. Blood cholesterol levels are affected by lack of exercise, a stressful lifestyle, the body's own mechanisms for production and excretion of cholesterol, and by diet. Accordingly, we can make food choices that help control our blood cholesterol levels.

Most advice that we hear seems to focus on limiting the amount of cholesterol in the diet. While this is important, it only provides one-fifth of the dietary solution to a very complicated problem. The other food factors that affect blood cholesterol are (1) excess fat, particularly saturated fat; (2) excess sugar; (3) inadequate fiber; and (4) excess calories.

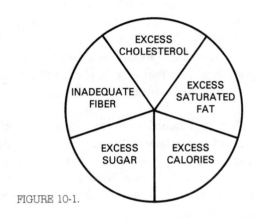

FIGURE 10-1.

Large amounts of saturated fat and sugar in the diet can increase blood cholesterol levels. Fiber-rich foods, on the other hand, help to decrease blood cholesterol levels. They decrease the absorption of cholesterol and saturated fat from the digestive system and increase their excretion from the body. Increased caloric intake is a problem if it leads to excess weight gain, since being overweight is also associated with elevated blood cholesterol levels.

Many of us have been led to believe that we can control our blood cholesterol level just by limiting the amount of eggs we eat. But this idea is not all it's cracked up to be. The solution is more complex than the elimination of any single food.

To continue to eat a diet low in fiber and high in saturated fat,

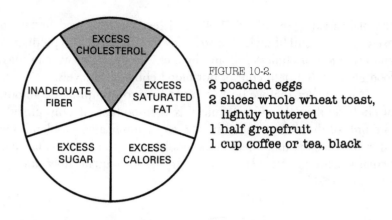

FIGURE 10-2.
2 poached eggs
2 slices whole wheat toast,
    lightly buttered
1 half grapefruit
1 cup coffee or tea, black

sugar, and calories, while avoiding eggs, is to put your eggs in the wrong basket. Eggs are a very nourishing food, and it makes little sense to exclude them from your diet. Nor is it wise to use a nutritionally inferior egg substitute. However, the manner in which eggs are eaten is, in fact, important.

A breakfast featuring an egg scrambled in plenty of butter, bacon or sausage, hash browns, and generously buttered toast is very high in saturated fat. Adding jam to the toast and sweetener to the coffee makes the meal high in sugar as well. Hence, what we do to the egg may well have more of a relationship to our blood cholesterol level than how the egg, alone, affects us.

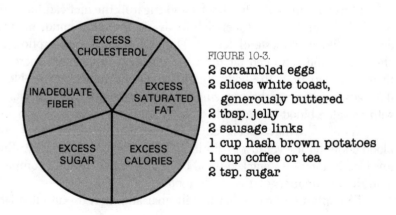

FIGURE 10-3.
2 scrambled eggs
2 slices white toast,
    generously buttered
2 tbsp. jelly
2 sausage links
1 cup hash brown potatoes
1 cup coffee or tea
2 tsp. sugar

TABLE 10-1. **Cholesterol in food.**

PORTION	FOOD	AVERAGE CHOLESTEROL (mg)
1	egg	250
1 ounce	liver, cooked	125
1 ounce	shrimp, cooked	40
1 cup	milk, whole	30
1 ounce	cheese, cheddar or jack	30
1 ounce	crab, lobster, cooked	25
1 ounce	beef, pork, lamb, cooked	25
1 ounce	poultry, cooked	25
1 ounce	fish, cooked	20
1 ounce	clams, oysters, cooked	20
1 teaspoon	butter	10
1 teaspoon	mayonnaise	5
1 teaspoon	margarine, vegetable oil	0
1 cup	legumes, cooked	0
1 handful	peanuts	0
1 cup	rice, oats, pasta, cooked	0
1 cup	fruit	0
1 cup	vegetable	0

You can see from Table 10-1 that cholesterol is found in all animal products, not just in eggs, but that it is not found in vegetable products. Note that one egg and a ten-ounce serving of meat have approximately the same amount of cholesterol. The meat, however, has about ten times more saturated fat. So, since saturated fat has also been implicated, along with dietary cholesterol, as a factor which influences blood cholesterol, it's best to cut down on meat consumption.

Contrary to popular belief, fish and poultry *do* contain cholesterol. However, they are very low in saturated fat. Shellfish, once thought to be high in cholesterol, really are not (with the possible exception of shrimp). In fact, since shellfish are so low in saturated fat, they are a healthy meal choice, provided they are not deep-fried or drenched in butter sauce.

In conclusion, the heart of the heart issue is to eat wholesome foods in moderation. Specifically, to help keep your blood cholesterol at a safe level,

1. Follow the suggestions in this book to
   - Decrease fat (especially saturated fat).
   - Decrease sugar.
   - Increase fiber-rich foods.
   - Modify calorie consumption to achieve and maintain ideal weight.
2. Reduce the cholesterol you eat by.
   - Limiting portions of meat, fish, poultry, and cheese to a combined total of 6 ounces daily.
     ○ Remember, each ounce of these foods contains about 25 milligrams of cholesterol.
     ○ See Chapter 8 for help in determining ounce equivalents for meat and cheese.
     ○ A chicken thigh or drumstick each contains about 2 ounces of meat, a wing about 1 ounce, and a breast about 3 ounces.
   - Limiting egg intake to an average of 6 weekly.
     ○ People with high blood cholesterol would be wise to restrict eggs to 3 or 4 weekly.
     ○ Egg restriction is unneccessary for premenopausal women, children, or vegetarians.

11

Shake Off
Your Salt Habit

Does your salting resemble a miniature blizzard? If it does, you may be cruising for trouble. Excess salt intake can lead to high blood pressure, a major risk factor for diseases of the cardiovascular system.

Of course, you need a certain amount of salt (specifically sodium) to maintain your fluid balance. But under normal conditions, there is no need to use a lot of salt since fresh foods contain sufficient sodium to keep your body functioning properly.

The salt shaker is not the only source of sodium. Fast foods and convenience foods are laced with salt and other sodium-containing compounds like sodium benzoate, monosodium glutamate, and sodium nitrate. Look at the difference between fresh and processed foods

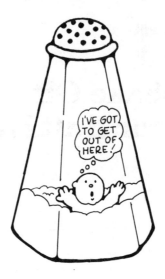

in Table 11-1. The next time you go shopping, see how many sodium substances you can find on labels of processed foods. We hope that you will be persuaded to buy fresh foods instead.

Shaking the salt habit is a wise move, especially if you have a family history of high blood pressure. In fact, cutting down on excessive salt intake while at the same time eating additional potassium-rich foods may be even more effective in controlling high blood pressure.

Here are some hints to get you started:

1. To decrease salt consumption,
    • Limit your intake of salty foods, including
        ○ Prepared soups (about 1 teaspoon of salt per can).
        ○ Potato chips, pretzels, salted nuts, and popcorn.
        ○ Condiments like soy sauce, steak sauce, and garlic salt.
        ○ Cheeses and pickled foods.
        ○ Cured meats like hot dogs and ham.
    • Use herbs and spices for flavor instead of salt.
    • Use garlic or onion powder rather than garlic or onion salt.

TABLE 11-1. **Sodium in fresh and processed foods.**

AMOUNT	FOOD	SODIUM (mg)
1 cup	milk, yogurt	120
1 oz.	cheddar, jack cheese	200
1/2 cup	cottage cheese	250
1 oz.	processed American cheese	325
1 oz.	processed cheese spread	455
1 oz.	processed American lowfat or low-cholesterol cheese	500
1 oz.	fresh meat, fish, poultry	25
1 oz.	ham	275
1 oz.	bologna, salami, pastrami	350
1	frankfurter	540
1	TV dinner	1100
1/2 cup	fresh vegetable	5
1/2 cup	canned vegetable	250
10	potato chips	75
1/2 cup	sauerkraut	560
1	black olive	75
1	green olive	150
1	dill pickle	1430
1/2 can	canned soup	1500
1 handful	unsalted peanuts	1
1 handful	salted peanuts	230
1/2 cup	cooked oatmeal, unsalted	1
1 oz.	shredded wheat	3
1/2 cup	cooked cereal, salted	280
1 oz.	cold cereal, containing salt	300
1 cup	rice or pasta, unsalted	1
1 cup	rice or pasta, salted	250
1 tsp.	salt, sea salt, seasoned salt	2300
1 tbsp.	soy sauce	1000
1 tsp.	MSG (Aćcent)	765
1 tsp.	herb, spice	trace
1 tsp.	butter or margarine, salted	50
1 tsp.	butter or margarine, unsalted	trace
1 tsp.	oil	trace

	BEANS	FISH	CHEESE	POULTRY	BEEF	LAMB	PORK	VEAL	EGGS	VEGETABLES	FRUIT	BREAD	SALAD
allspice		x		x	x	x		x			x	x	
basil		x							x	x			x
bay leaf	x	x		x	x	x		x					
cardamom											x	x	
celery seed		x	x		x	x	x	x		x			
chervil			x		x	x	x	x	x	x			x
cinnamon						x					x	x	
cloves				x	x		x	x			x	x	
chili	x			x	x		x		x				
cumin	x		x	x					x			x	
dill weed		x								x		x	x
ginger				x	x		x	x			x	x	
marjoram	x	x		x	x	x	x	x	x	x			x
mustard	x	x	x	x				x					x
nutmeg			x								x	x	
oregano	x	x	x	x	x	x	x	x	x	x			x
parsley	x	x	x	x	x	x	x	x	x	x			x
rosemary		x		x	x	x	x	x					
sage				x	x	x	x	x					
savory		x		x	x	x	x	x	x				x
sesame seed		x	x	x						x		x	x
tarragon		x		x	x	x	x		x				x
thyme		x	x	x	x	x	x	x	x	x			x

FIGURE 11-1. **A guide to the spice islands.**

- Decrease salt in your recipes to half, or better, to a quarter, of the suggested amount.
- Do not automatically salt cooking water; use a bay leaf for flavor instead.
- Try to add less than ½ teaspoon salt to food daily.

2. To increase potassium intake, use the following potassium-rich foods:
   - All fruits (not just bananas and oranges).
   - Fresh and frozen vegetables, but not canned vegetables because they have salt added.
   - Grains, particularly those prepared with little or no salt (for example, oatmeal, rice, and noodles).
   - Legumes (beans, peas, and lentils).
   - Unsalted nuts and seeds.

A variety of seasonings used to enhance the flavors of common foods can be found in Figure 11-1. Those herbs and spices that go well with each particular food are noted by an *x* in each column. Do not put all the suggested seasonings into one dish. Rather, experiment with one or several at a time to create a variety of tastes from the same basic food. Check out the recipe section to see how these seasonings are used.

> *Your salt intake should be less.*
> *Foods with spices and herbs, bless.*
>
> *Garlic, onion, lemon, wine*
> *Make your dishes really fine.*
>
> *Get in that kitchen and create*
> *Foods that look and taste real great.*
>
> *On these hints you should now mull*
> *So that your meals will not be dull!*

12
What's Brewing?

Are you a zombie until your morning coffee? If so, you are hooked on the most popular stimulant in the world—caffeine. Coffee supplies most of the caffeine that we ingest, but tea, chocolate, and cola beverages also contribute substantial amounts, as do a variety of medications. Check Table 12-1 to find out how much caffeine you consume each day.

A moderate amount of caffeine, like that present in one or two cups of coffee, may be just the thing to perk you up. However, when you plug yourself into a continual flow of caffeine all day long, other effects begin to brew.

Ingestion of 200 milligrams of caffeine or more is associated with sleeplessness, irritability, and nervousness. Some heavy-caffeine users have actually been treated for anxiety neurosis. Digestive disturbances,

TABLE 12-1. **Caffeine in selected foods, beverages, and drugs.***

FOOD/BEVERAGE/DRUG	SERVING	CAFFEINE (mg)
Chocolate bar	1 oz.	20
Cocoa (hot chocolate)	8 oz.	13
Coffee		
Instant	5 oz.	62
Percolated	5 oz.	102
Dripolated	5 oz.	136
Cola and soda beverages		
Coca Cola	12 oz.	65
Dr Pepper	12 oz.	61
Mountain Dew	12 oz.	55
Tab	12 oz.	49
Pepsi	12 oz.	43
Tea, black		
5-minute brew	5 oz.	46
1-minute brew	5 oz.	28
Nonprescription drugs		
Anacin	tab	32
Aspirin Compound	tab	32
Bromo-Seltzer	tab	32
Cope	tab	32
Easy-Mens	tab	32
Emperin Compound	tab	32
Excedrin	tab	60
Midol	tab	32
No-Doze	tab	100
Pre-Mens	tab	66
Vanquish	tab	42
Many cold preparations	tab	30
Many stimulants	tab	100
Prescription drugs		
APC	tab	32
Carergot	tab	100
Darvon	tab	32
Fiorinal	tab	40
Migral	tab	50

*Based on Bunker, 1979; Stephenson, 1977.

particularly hyperacid stomach and heartburn, appear to be associated as much with decaffeinated as with regular coffee.

Caffeine also affects the cardiovascular system by raising the blood pressure and resting heart rate, and it can even cause an abnormal heart rhythm in susceptible people.

Recent research suggests that caffeine, and caffeine-like substances known as xanthines, may aggravate fibrocystic breast disease. Elimination of coffee, tea, chocolate, and cola from the diet appears to decrease significantly the swelling and tenderness characteristic of this disease.

Keep in mind that dose is related to body size. A child drinking a 12-ounce can of cola gets proportionately as much caffeine as an adult who drinks four cups of coffee. Restlessness, nervousness, and irritability in children may thus be related more to beverage ingestion than to disposition. Caffeine also passes through the placenta and into breast milk, possibly affecting the fetus and the nursing infant.

The way you drink your caffeinated beverage may be interfering with your plans for "girth" control. Each teaspoon of sugar adds about 20 empty calories to your cup of coffee or tea, while a tablespoon of cream adds another 40. Ten cups a day can add anywhere from zero to over a thousand calories, depending on how sweet and light you like it. Remember also that the average can of caffeine-containing soda contains about 150 calories.

In summary, caffeine can offer a reasonable solution to the problem of momentary fatigue. Caffeine, however, is a drug, and in large doses may be harmful to certain sensitive individuals. To avoid problems, it's best to keep caffeine consumption from all sources below 200 milligrams a day. There's no harm in avoiding it altogether, but if you are considering cold-turkey withdrawal, be aware that such a drastic change may cause headaches for awhile. A gradual withdrawal from caffeine will be easier on your head and the psyche inside it.

If you "urn" your way through the day, here are some decaffeinating techniques.

1. Drink smaller cups or dilute the coffee with half a cup of warm milk. Milk is naturally sweet, so you won't need to add sugar.

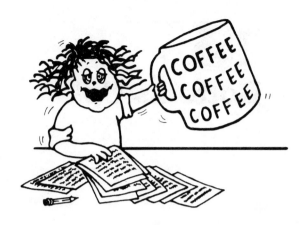

2. Between meals, substitute a cup of water for every other cup of coffee, tea, or cola you usually drink. Gradually begin to choose water more frequently.

3. Substitute decaffeinated coffee, Pero, Postum, or herbal tea, particularly in the evening.

   • Note: It's best not to use decaffeinated coffee excessively, as it still contains substances that irritate the stomach.

   • Also, several herbal teas are made with maté or guarana, which contain caffeine.

4. Try hot lemon tea for a quick pickup. Just stir the juice from half a lemon and a teaspoon of sugar or honey into a cup of boiling water. Refreshing!

5. Prepare only enough coffee or tea so that you can savor one or two cups when it's freshly brewed. Throw away any leftovers to avoid temptation.

6. Try some stretching exercises or a five-minute walk rather than coffee to perk you up.

   • Your trips to the coffee pot may reflect your need for a change of pace, rather than a real desire for more caffeine.

   • In fact, the act of going to get the coffee might actually be more refreshing than drinking it.

13
Bottoms Up!

Have you ever been polluted? You know, that awful feeling after having had a few too many. Your body and head feel as if they've been run over by a steamroller. This rarely happens after just one drink; a little alcohol can be enjoyable, but too much can be disastrous. The amount of alcohol you drink determines whether you're building a healthy or polluted environment within your body.

Because they're high in calories and contain a minimal amount of essential nutrients, alcoholic beverages are a kind of adult junk food. Spirited beverages contain about 150 calories in their most commonly consumed sizes: a 12-ounce can of beer; an 8-ounce glass of wine; a 2-ounce shot of hard liquor. This alone is a good reason to go easy on these beverages. Social drinkers often gain weight because of their drinks and the munchies that they eat with them.

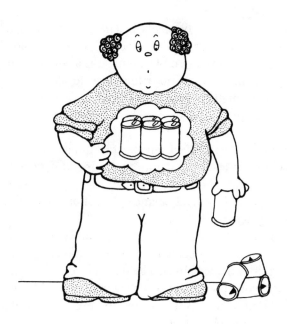

Most of the alcohol we drink cannot fuel muscle or brain power directly. Ninety percent of it goes to the liver where it is metabolized (changed into energy) at a slow, constant rate. Processing only small amounts of alcohol at a time, the liver needs about two hours to metabolize the alcohol in a 12-ounce can of beer, a 6-ounce glass of wine or a 1½-ounce jigger of hard liquor. Once you start consuming alcoholic beverages faster than this, your blood levels of alcohol begin to get high and so do you.

If you've had one too many, the usual attempts to sober up (coffee, cold showers, walking it off) may stimulate your nervous system so you feel more awake. But these methods decrease neither the amount of alcohol in your body nor the damage it is doing; you can be wide awake and drunk at the same time. Remember, only time and your liver can get rid of the alcohol.

Bigger people, because of their larger bloodstreams, can accomodate slightly more alcohol than their lightweight friends. That's why the average woman gets tipsy before her male counterpart, though they consume the same amount of alcohol. The presence of food in the stomach slows the rate with which alcohol enters the bloodstream. Thus, drinking rapidly on an empty stomach is a sure way to get high quickly. Heavy drinkers build up a tolerance to alcohol, so it takes more to make them high. Being able to "hold one's liquor," then, may be more an indicator of liver damage and alcoholism, than a sign of being "cool."

Because of its adverse effects on appetite and the digestive system, excessive alcohol use leads to vitamin and mineral deficiencies. Furthermore, the diuretic action of alcohol can lead to severe disturbances in the body's fluid and mineral balance. Nutritional anemias are also common among heavy drinkers.

Alcohol is directly toxic to the liver, the nervous system, and the heart. Excess amounts can decrease your body's ability to build protein, slowing the repair of tissue damaged by normal wear and tear. Alcohol can also impair your power to learn new and store old information. Antibody production, too, is diminished by excessive drinking, lessening your ability to fight infection.

Gastrointestinal disturbances can result from drinking too much alcohol. These problems include indigestion, stomach trouble, hepatitis, pancreatitis, cirrhosis, and malabsorption of many nutrients. Excess alcohol can also damage the lining of your mouth, throat, stomach, and intestine. Cancer of the throat and neck is much more common in people who drink than in people who do not, especially for those who also smoke. In pregnant women, excessive alcohol intake leads to irreversible damage to the fetus; two drinks daily is the limit for expectant mothers. In men, too much alcohol can cause impotence.

Though excessive alcohol is definitely unhealthy for your body and your mind, small amounts may actually be good for you. It seems that teetotalers do not live as long as those who drink occasionally. Recent studies show that a few drinks weekly may decrease your risk of heart disease. Once alcohol accounts for 20 percent or more of your average daily calories, however, you may be setting yourself up for serious trouble. (An average of three servings of wine, beer, or hard liquor daily supplies about 20 percent of 2000 calories.)

Here are some strategies to help you fight body pollution.

1. Limit yourself to one, perhaps two, drinks a day or less.
2. Make sure that you have eaten or are eating something while you drink.
3. If you are pregnant, try to avoid alcohol altogether. It's doubtful, however, that an occasional drink will hurt.
4. Alternate alcoholic with nonalcoholic beverages. Perrier water or club soda with a twist is refreshing and has become a popular substitute for mixed drinks.
5. Choose a beverage that's not your favorite. The best-liked drinks seem to go down the fastest.
6. Try to avoid sweetened mixers.
   • Aside from adding extra sugar and calories, they also mask the bitter taste of alcohol, a natural deterrent to excess drinking.
   • Having your drink straight up may actually help to slow you down.
7. Forget about the "one for the road."
   • Try winding down your drinking an hour or so before you leave for home.
   • Linger over a warm beverage and conversation, allowing your liver time to use the booze you've already imbibed.
8. If you are hosting a party, make sure that there are plenty of nonalcoholic beverages readily available. Many of your guests will be pleased to have an alternative.
9. If you are a guest, tote along some nonalcoholic beverages to your next BYOB party.

14

When You're Weigh Off Balance

Holding on to that perfect weight is a balancing act. Given individual differences in metabolism, we each must find that balance of energy intake and output that brings us to our ideal weight and keeps us there. This is no easy task in our sedentary food-filled world. Yet maintenance of ideal weight is extremely important because excessive weight is a major risk factor for cancer, diabetes, high blood pressure, strokes, and heart disease. Besides, many people view overweight as being unattractive. But whether for good health or good looks, fat is something we should not be.

The popularity of reducing plans, diet books, and slenderizing gadgetry is proof enough that we do have a big problem. Every month there is a new fad diet, and yet we abandon these diets as quickly as we begin them. Nutritionally disastrous, they are also boring, rigid, and difficult to fit into any reasonable lifestyle. Our efforts at weight control, inspired by "monthly miracle plans," produce short-term deprivation, temporary weight loss, and guilt that results from weight rapidly regained. Because they fail to reshape our behaviors and attitudes about the calories we eat and expend, fad diets could accurately be dubbed "Regimes That Lose At Losing."

Winning at weight loss is not impossible, but it does require a commitment, though not as great a commitment as you may think. Fad diets fail because they demand that the dieter be an unabashed, superhuman masochist. To take the "die" out of dieting, make a small commitment for a long time. It works.

Consider that 3,500 calories make a pound. If your goal is to lose a pound a week, you will need to create a daily deficit of 500 calories. You won't see a rapid drop in your weight, but you will notice small, steady losses that will produce big results in the long run.

Because exercise is vital for your body, mind, and soul, it should be included in any weight-control plan. Of course, you can instead

---

Deficit Spending Can Avoid Inflation of Your Fat Mass

You can eat less
- Cut your 8-ounce meat portion down to 4 ounces — 300
- Use 1 tablespoon of salad dressing instead of
  3 tablespoons — 150
- Make your regular beer a light brew — 70
  — 520

You can exercise more
- Do one hour of jogging or aerobic dance — 600

Eat a little less and do a little more:
- Cut your 8-ounce meat portion in half — 300
- Jog for 20 minutes
  (How's that?!) — 200
  — 500

---

decrease your food intake drastically, but in so doing you will jeopardize your health and feel crummy. This is hardly a practical or healthful idea. The rewards that come with a sensible diet and exercise will help you stick to your guns. Moderation is really the key to motivation.

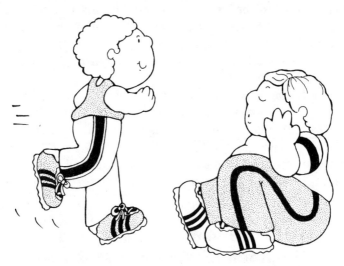

You should also be aware that small snacks can have a cumulative effect on your weight and yield big results you don't need. A raid on the refrigerator for a munch or drink of 100 calories extra each day adds up to a yearly 36,500 calories. Zap! Ten extra pounds. This weight gain is insidious, though, because at 100 extra calories a day you gain only about three ounces each week. A half-hour daily walk, on the other hand, could help you burn 67,700 calories a year—18 pounds worth! You see, it's the little things you do (or don't do) each day that determine whether the bathroom scale is the bearer of good news.

Affecting the calories you eat and use are other powerful influences, namely your behavior around food and your attitude about your weight. These factors make weight control something more complex than a simple measurement of calories in or out! If you are overweight, "calories" are an intellectual thing but "eating" is an emotional affair. You need to become sensitive to the feelings you have that undermine your ability to lose weight.

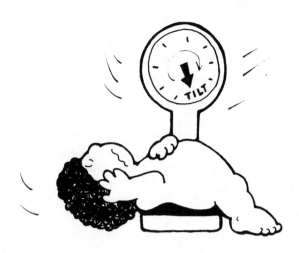

Several outstanding books on weight control are included in the Suggested Reading List (see Appendix C). They are loaded with suggestions to help you maintain a thinner lifestyle. A starter set of behavioral suggestions follows, or you may wish to follow "The Slimmer Weigh."

Fight Fat Ten Ways

1.   Eat slowly. Chew a lot. Gulping won't make you gorgeous.

2.   Make your portions small and take only one helping (except for vegetables). You'll get a chance to eat your favorite foods again.

3.   Beware of your emotions. If you're reaching for food to make you content or relaxed, don't be fooled! Extra food usually doesn't calm you down. Because it adds extra pounds, it may even make you more upset.

4.   What turns you on to food? Wait for a hunger pang. If you can't remember what one feels like, you're eating off cue. Many of us eat from habit, not from hunger.

5.   Beware of raids on the refrigerator. Get the goodies out of the house, since they are baddies for you.

6. Watch where and how you eat. Eat at the table sitting on a chair. Watch out for automatic eating—at the movies, in front of the TV, while you're reading. Do you really need all the food you are carting around from place to place? Remember, if it's excessive, you'll be carting it around in the form of a padded body.

7. Don't be pressured into eating just to be socially acceptable. At parties choose low-calorie foods. Don't stand next to the food table. If you find you're suffering from "hand to mouth" syndrome, sit on your hands or assist the host.

8. Don't let yourself be intimidated by weak-willed dieters. They'll envy your ability to change your eating habits.

9. Sit less. Do more. Getting fat is easy if you don't move. Use up some energy. Find an activity that's fun and do it regularly.

10. Put some pleasure in your life. Reward yourself with something other than food: a new record album, a trip to the theater, a long-distance phone call to an old friend. These won't cause the remorse that high-caloried splurges usually do!

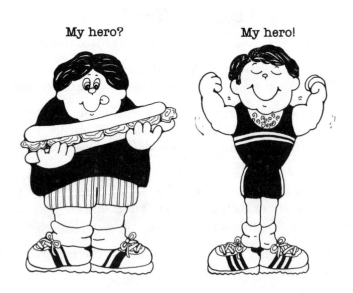

My hero?　　　　My hero!

The Slimmer Weigh

Shop Slim
1. Make a list and stick to it.
2. Include only nutritious foods.
   - Lean meats, poultry, fish, legumes.
   - Whole-grain breads and cereals.
   - Lowfat dairy products.
   - Plenty of colorful fruits and vegetables.
3. Shop on a full stomach to avoid impulsive buying of high-calorie foods.

Cook Slim/Eat Slim
1. Reduce fat (see Chapter 8).
2. Avoid sugar and refined foods (see Chapters 4 and 6).
3. Prepare plenty of bulky foods.
   - At least one fruit at (or between) each meal.
   - At least two vegetables at lunch and dinner.

Drink Slim
1. Quench thirst with water.
2. Drink coffee and tea "straight."
3. Avoid sweetened juices and drinks.
   - In fact, go easy on all juices, sweetened or not.
   - Just think—one cup of apple juice has the same calories as three apples!
4. Watch out at cocktail time.
   - 5-ounce glass of table wine   85 calories
   - 1 1/2-ounce jigger of hard liquor   110 calories
   - 1 mixed drink   160 calories
   - 12-ounce can of beer   160 calories

Act Slim
1. Take the time to sit down and enjoy your meals.
2. Eat slowly. Chew a lot.

3. When you eat, only eat. Avoid other activities like reading, talking on the phone, etc.
4. Increase your physical activity.
   - 20 minutes of brisk aerobic activity will burn up 150 to 250 calories.
   - Try brisk walking, dancing, jogging, swimming, biking, racketball, basketball, or tennis.
   - The important thing is that you find some activity you really like to do and then do a bit every day.
5. Develop new interests, hobbies, and skills to add interest to your life.

Think Slim

1. Be patient with yourself and your weight loss.
   - Remember, it takes awhile to learn new eating and exercise habits.
   - Also, a loss of two pounds per week is the maximum recommended in order for you to remain healthy.
2. Plan for occasional treats as *part of* your weight control program.
   - This helps you not to feel so "deprived."
   - An infrequent foray into high-cal foods is not a disaster. It's what you do 80 percent of the time that *really* counts.
   - And, if you're going to "blow it," blow it on quality food. Make those calories count, if not for nutrition, then at least for taste.
3. Think positive thoughts.
   - Negative thoughts about yourself and your weight work against you.
   - Accept yourself as you are and visualize yourself becoming slimmer.

Stay Slim

1. Realize that weight control is a long-term process, not something you do for a while. "Going on a diet" implies going off it, too.
2. Engage in physical activity regularly.
   - Exercise helps you lose weight faster and maintain your loss more easily.

- Exercise also has a calming effect, making it less likely that you will eat out of frustration.
3. Measure and weigh yourself weekly.
   - The measurements are important because you may be getting smaller, yet see no appreciable difference in your weight.
   - That's because you are losing fat but gaining muscle.

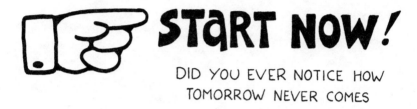

START NOW!

DID YOU EVER NOTICE HOW
TOMORROW NEVER COMES

15
Do It
with Groups

If you've ever counted calories you know how tedious it can be. The "exchange system" is a method that simplifies the process. The system divides foods into the following six groups:

1. Milk Exchanges
2. Vegetable Exchanges
3. Fruit Exchanges
4. Bread Exchanges
5. Meat Exchanges
6. Fat Exchanges

Foods within each group are nutritionally and calorically similar, so that specified amounts of each can be "exchanged" for another. For example, one small orange and half a grapefruit equal one fruit exchange each. If your breakfast calls for one exchange (serving) of fruit, you can choose either the orange or the grapefruit half; either choice provides approximately 40 calories, most of these from carbohydrates. Thus, when you think in terms of eating a specific number of servings from each group, you accomplish two things at once; you plan for specific caloric level, and you plan for a nutritionally balanced diet.

Get to know the foods in each group by referring to the Exchange System in Appendix A. Underline or asterisk your favorites and note the serving size. Break out your measuring spoons and cups and measure your foods for several days. Soon you'll be able to "eyeball" the right amount of food. While it isn't necessary to measure everything you eat forever, it is a good idea to learn what other foods equal a half cup of cereal, a teaspoon of butter, etc. A small scale helps if you want to measure cooked portions of meat.

If you plan to use the exchange system, see Table 15-1 for the recommended combinations of food groups to help you meet your nutrient requirements. Three different plans are listed: 1200 calories, 1500 calories, and 1800 calories. Alongside each calorie level is listed the number of servings recommended from each group of food. By following the suggested number of servings given, you will automatically limit your fat intake to 30% of your total calories. If you eat less than 1500 calories a day, it's a good idea to take a low-potency multiple vitamin and mineral supplement daily (see Chapter 19 for more information).

Small, frequent meals are more effective for weight reduction than one huge meal at the end of the day. When you spread your

TABLE 15-1. **Sample weight-loss plans.**

TOTAL CALORIES	MILK	VEGETABLE	FRUIT	BREAD	MEAT	FAT
	Servings	Servings	Servings	Servings	Servings	Servings
1200	1	3	3	6	4	6
1500	1 1/2	4	4	7	5	8
1800	2	5	4	9	6	9

TABLE 15-2. **1200-calorie sample menu.**

BREAKFAST:	
1 cup cooked oats	2 Bread
1 cup lowfat milk	1 Milk + 1 Fat
2 tbsp. raisins	1 Fruit
2 tsp. sunflower seeds	1 Fat
LUNCH:	
1 slice cheddar cheese	1 Meat + 1 Fat
1/4 cup tuna	1 Meat
1 tsp. mayonnaise	1 Fat
2 slice whole-grain bread	2 Bread
1/2 cup tomatoes	1 Vegetable
Lettuce, parsley, radishes	Free
SNACK:	
1 orange	1 Fruit
DINNER:	
2 oz. baked chicken (with herbs)	2 Meat
Fat-free meat juice	Free
1 large baked potato	2 Bread
2 tbsp. sour cream	1 Fat
Chives	Free
1/2 cup steamed broccoli	1 Vegetable
1 tbsp. Italian dressing	1 Fat
Deep green leafy lettuce, parsley	Free
1/4 cup tomatoes	1/2 Vegetable
1/4 cup grated carrots	1/2 Vegetable
SNACK:	
3/4 cup strawberries	1 Fruit
2 tbsp. sour cream (thinned with 1 tbsp. buttermilk)	1 Fat

meals throughout the day, you can plan for at least three meals and still have room for snacks. To give you a better idea, look at the "1200-Calorie Sample Menu" (Table 15-2), which features three meals plus two snacks.

To design your own low-calorie scheme, use the 1200-calorie meal plan from Table 15-1 as a foundation. Remember, you can reduce fat and increase fiber by eating lean or light meats and heavy dark breads, as well as by including fruits and vegetables with each meal.

A healthy dinner looks like this.

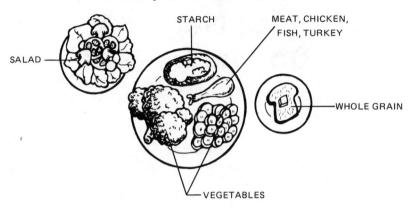

Not like this.

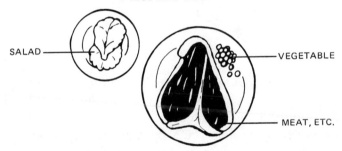

16

Dining Out
Need Not
Do You In

Eating out is an integral part of today's lifestyle. But this doesn't mean that it's impossible for you to be discriminating about the foods you choose in a restaurant. Don't use dining out as a psychological subterfuge to allow you to eat indiscriminately, or you will undermine all your good intentions; be aware of these "Pitfalls at the Pitstop":

1. *I'm paying for it, so I may as well finish it.*
   - If you're eating on an expense account, you're kidding yourself.
   - Leave part of your portion behind.
   - Take part home in a doggie bag and eat the rest tomorrow.
   - Share your entree with someone else.

2. *Just this once won't hurt.*
    • This is true if just this once is a rare happening.
    • A lot of "just this onces" can do you in.
3. *Poor me, I deserve a treat.*
    • Is frequent fattening fare really a treat?
    • Find some nonfood "uppers" when you're down.
    • If you're traveling for business, try filling up some lonely hours on the road with a long walking exploration around town, a run, or a workout at a gym.
4. *I should not waste this food.*
    • Your choice—waist or waste.
    • There is no way starving children benefit from the food *you* eat!
5. *I've already blown it today. I'll start again next week.*
    • One meal never made anyone fat.
    • Poor attitude. Waiting around could mean waisting around.

To help you carry out your new program, refer to the following "Insights into Initiating Innovations in Eateries":

1. Plan *where* you will eat.
    • Pick a place with a varied menu where you feel comfortable with the alternatives.
2. Plan *what* you will eat.
    • Figure out if it's time for poultry, fish, or meat before you ever get there.
    • Then, stick to your guns when ordering.
3. Plan *how much* you will eat.
    • If you're going to a restaurant where the portions are large, decide ahead that you will eat only part of the serving.

If you usually eat out at lunch, consider brown-bagging it on occasion. That way you can include the foods that are difficult to find in restaurants, like fresh fruits and whole-grain breads. When traveling, try to have a whole-grain cereal like oatmeal or shredded wheat for breakfast. Lunches are a good time to include a large salad for extra fiber. Easy on the dressing, though.

When scanning a menu, focus on the better alternatives. The following "Menu Confrontation" list is a guide to "Easy Eyeballing to Eliminate Endangered Eating":

1. *First Courses*
   - Go with fruit, juice, or consommé.
2. *Salads*
   - Ask for dressing on the side. If your salad comes dressed, it may be wearing 500 calories!
3. *Entrees*
   - Steer clear of fried foods and those in cream sauces. The four B's save calories—bake, broil, boil, and barbecue.
   - Go with light meats often—fish, poultry, or veal (not breaded). If you eat steak, choose a filet mignon, flank steak, or sirloin; they're quite lean compared to other cuts.
4. *Accompaniments*
   - Request a substitution (sliced tomatoes, for example) for fried potatoes.
   - Baked potatoes are great, but watch what you put on them. Two tablespoons of sour cream contain the same amount of calories and fat as one teaspoon of butter.
5. *Desserts*
   - Potential disaster zone. Order fruit if you can, or taste a bit of someone else's dessert.

Note the differences between typical restaurant choices and more discriminating choices in Table 16-1. Each *F* represents a teaspoon of fat. High-fiber foods are circled.

TABLE 16-1. **Restaurant menu selection.**

TYPICAL CHOICE		BETTER CHOICE	
2 fried eggs	FFF	½ GRAPEFRUIT	
4 links sausage	FFFF	1 CUP OATMEAL	
1 cup hash browns	FFF	1 cup whole milk	FF
3 coffees with cream		1 SLICE WHOLE WHEAT	
and sugar	FFF	TOAST	
		1 pat butter	F
		1 poached egg	F
		1 black coffee	
Diet Plate with:		1/2 cup juice	
8 oz. ground beef	FFFF	3 oz. turkey on	F
	FFFF	2 SLICES WHOLE WHEAT	
1/2 cup cottage cheese	F	1 tsp. mayonnaise	F
2 peach halves		SLICED TOMATOES	
1/2 cup jello		1 FRESH ORANGE	
2 pkg. melba toast		1 black coffee	
2 coffees with cream			
and sugar	FF		
2 martinis		1 martini	
SALAD		SALAD	
2 ladles blue cheese	FFFFFF	1/2 ladle Italian	
dressing	FFFFFF	dressing	FF
2 slices french bread		1 SLICE WHOLE WHEAT	
4 pats butter	FFFF	BREAD	
10 oz. steak	FFFFF	1 pat butter	F
	FFFFF	5 oz. filet mignon	FFF
1 BAKED POTATO		1 BAKED POTATO	
1/4 cup sour cream	FF	2 tbsp. sour cream	F
12 oz. wine		4 oz. wine	
2 coffees with cream		1 black coffee	
and sugar	FF		
Total calories	5022	Total calories	1886
Calories fat	2997	Calories fat	630
% calories fat	60%	% calories fat	33%

17

May the Source Be with You

Don't go without the source—that is, the source of needed nutrients. There are some nutrients that you may not be getting in sufficient quantity in your daily diet, such as folic acid, vitamins B-6, C, and E, calcium, magnesium, potassium, iron, selenium, and zinc. If you follow all the suggestions given in this book, your diet will include foods rich in these vitamins and minerals.

To ensure maximum nutrient retention during food preparation, it's best to wash and cut fresh vegetables immediately before cooking. Leave the skins on whenever possible. (Your friends and family will get used to mashed potatoes with flecks of brown skin in them. They're actually more tasty that way.) Stir-fry, steam, or cook vegetables tightly covered in a minimal amount of boiling water until crispy-tender. This usually takes only about five or ten minutes. Save the vegetable cooking water and use it in sauces, soups, or as a beverage with your meal.

If you use frozen vegetables, be sure not to let them thaw before cooking, as nutrients will be lost. Instead, place frozen vegetables directly into a small amount of boiling water, cover tightly, and boil briefly. Remember, frozen vegetables have already been partially cooked (blanched), so they need very little additional cooking. Frozen vegetables can also be stir-fried in a bit of oil, though they will not have the flavor or crunch of fresh vegetables cooked in this manner. For more information on foods rich in some key nutrients, consult Tables 17-1 and 17-2.

TABLE 17-1. **Food sources of selected vitamins.**

FOLIC ACID	VITAMIN B-6	VITAMIN C	VITAMIN E
Asparagus	Bananas	Broccoli	Avocados
Beet greens	Dark green	Brussel	Legumes
Bok choy	leafy	sprouts	Nuts and seeds
Broccoli	vegetables	Cabbage	Peanuts and
Brussel sprouts	Egg yolk	Cauliflower	peanut butter
Cabbage	Fish and	Citrus fruits	Vegetable oils
Chard	shellfish	Dark green	(particularly
Cilantro	Legumes	leafy	safflower)
Mint	Muscle	vegetables	Whole-grain
Parsley	meats,	Melons	breads and
Red leaf lettuce	liver, and	Peppers,	cereals
Romaine lettuce	kidney	green or	
Scallions	Peanuts,	chili	
Spinach	peanut	Strawberries	
Watercress	butter,	Tomatoes	
	walnuts,		
	and filberts		
	Potatoes and		
	sweet		
	potatoes		
	Prunes and		
	raisins		
	Whole-grain		
	breads and		
	cereals		
	Yeast		

TABLE 17-2. Food sources of selected minerals.

CALCIUM	IRON	MAGNESIUM	POTASSIUM	SELENIUM	ZINC
Canned fish (salmon, sardines, mackerel)	Blackstrap molasses	Bananas	Fruits	Fish	Cheeses
Cheeses	Dark green leafy vegetables	Dark green leafy vegetables	Legumes	Garlic	Legumes
Dark green leafy vegetables	Dried fruits	Legumes	Nuts and seeds	Kidney	Meat
Dried fruit	Iron cooking utensils	Nuts	Vegetables, fresh and frozen	Meat	Nuts and seeds
Milk	Legumes	Peanuts and peanut butter	Whole-grain breads and cereals	Mushrooms	Shellfish
Tofu (soy curd)	Liver	Whole-grain breads and cereals		Whole-grain breads and cereals	Whole-grain breads and cereals
Yogurt	Red meat			Yeast (if grown on selenium-rich food)	
	Whole-grain breads and cereals				

18
Shopping Around

For the most part, all the foods you need to eat are already in your local food store. If you examine the layout of a typical market, you will probably find that the fresh foods are usually placed around the perimeter of the store, while the canned, boxed, and instant foods fill the center shelves. You can actually zip around the outer aisles and buy just about everything you need. An occasional trip into the interior will give you a chance to stock up on cereal, pasta, tuna, tomato sauce, and dry goods. For more information on finding nourishing foods in your local market, read *The Supermarket Handbook* (see the Recommended Reading List in Appendix C).

An occasional trip to a health food store might be a good idea. There you'll find a wider variety of whole-grain products, including whole-wheat pasta. You can buy from bulk bins, which helps reduce

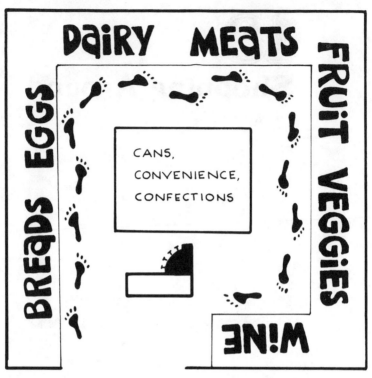

FOLLOW FEET FOR FAST SHOPPING!!!

the cost of some items. Frequently, foods in these stores cost a great deal more than those available at the local markets. So compare value and taste and decide which you prefer. But be judicious in choosing health foods, too. Just because it's in a health food store, doesn't necessarily mean that a food is healthy. High-fat, high-sugar foods can be labeled "natural," too.

19

To 'B' or Not To 'B': A Supplementary Note

Do you need to take vitamin and/or mineral supplements? If you are healthy and not overstressed, the answer to this question is "no," provided you regularly eat a variety of fresh and underprocessed foods.

Unfortunately, if you are a typical American, you probably don't eat this way. In fact, the average American now gets nearly half of his daily calories from highly refined fats, sweeteners, and alcohol. As is explained earlier in this book, these highly refined products supply mainly empty calories, those without the vitamins, minerals, protein, and fiber that are present in the foods from which they are derived.

Therefore, you may benefit from the extra "insurance" of a low-potency, well-balanced multiple vitamin and mineral supplement, particularly if you fit into one or several of the following categories:

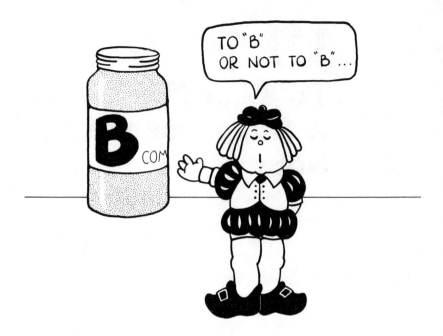

1. Eat out frequently.
2. Rely on fast foods or highly processed convenience foods much of the time.
3. Munch on high-fat and high-sugar snacks often.
4. Skip meals regularly.
5. Go on and off diets in an effort to control weight.
6. Routinely eat very little.
   - Less than 1500 calories for those over 11 years old.
   - Less than 1000 calories for children 4 to 10 years old.
   - Less than 900 calories for infants 2 to 3 years old.
7. Have an illness, anemia, injury, or are recovering from either of these.
8. Take medications daily.

It's important to choose a multiple vitamin and mineral supplement that contains those nutrients that are not usually added back to processed foods. These include vitamins E and B-6, folic acid, biotin, pantothenic acid, magnesium, zinc, copper, chromium, and selenium. Biotin is actually made by the bacteria in your digestive tract. However, these organisms can be destroyed by antibiotics. Therefore, taking a supplement containing biotin is beneficial if you have to rely on antibiotic therapy over a long period of time. To compare available formulas with a guide based on the 1980 Recommended Dietary Allowances, see Appendix B. Available products most closely resembling these recommendations are also listed there.

Buying bottles containing a single nutrient is not a wise idea, because taking too much of one nutrient can increase your need for one or several others. Besides, it's costly. Be careful of using very large doses of supplemental vitamins and minerals. This is particularly true of vitamins A and D, as well as of the trace minerals like iron, zinc, copper, iodine, chromium, and selenium. Stick with a low-potency, well-balanced multiple.

Supplements are most effective when taken with meals because food aids in their absorption and use by the body. Also, a few smaller doses are absorbed more effectively than one large dose. Therefore, a multiple vitamin and mineral supplement with the daily dose broken into two or three tablets is the most beneficial—for those who can remember to take them.

You may have heard that "natural" supplements are better than the so-called synthetic or man-made varieties. Actually, the only supplements that can really be considered natural are those made solely from food concentrates (see Table 19-1). Just like the foods from which they are derived, concentrates are composed of several nutrients that work together for optimum use by the body. Supplements made purely from food concentrates are low-potency and usually more expensive than supplements containing synthetic vitamins.

It turns out that most so-called natural supplements contain some synthetic vitamins in a base of food concentrate. The amount of the food concentrate may actually be very small. The synthetic vitamin is added to increase potency so that a lot of vitamin can be squeezed into a small pill. This also helps to keep the price reasonable.

The only truly natural vitamins are found in food. It is extremely

TABLE 19-1.

FOOD CONCENTRATES	NUTRIENTS SUPPLIED
Fish oils	Vitamins A and D.
Nutritional or brewer's yeast	Vitamin B-complex, as well as chromium and selenium (if grown on compound rich in these minerals); torula yeast is a poor source of chromium.
Citrus, rose hips, acerola cherries	Vitamin C.
Wheat germ oil	Vitamin E.
Oyster shells, egg shells, bone meal	Calcium and magnesium, as well as phosphorus; since bone meal may be contaminated with lead, it's best not to use supplements which contain it.
Kelp	Iodine and other trace minerals.

important to remember that adding supplements to a diet overrich in coffee, alcohol, sugar, fat, and salt cannot reverse the damage done by excess amounts of any of these. Supplements can never take the place of a healthy diet of fresh, unrefined, and underprocessed foods.

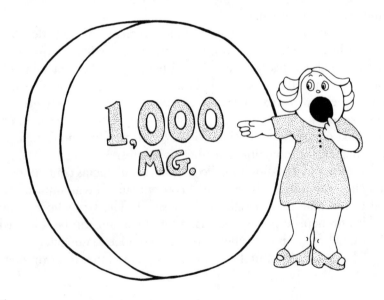

Recipes

On the pages that follow you will find some of our favorite recipes featuring fresh, whole, and underprocessed ingredients. In these dishes you can enjoy the delicate and delicious flavor of foods prepared with a minimum of fat, sugar, and salt.

The recipes encourage the use of poultry, veal, fish, and beans. This will help you reduce the saturated fat content of your diet so that you can use a small amount of butter if you wish. Whole grains and vegetables are suggested as accompaniments, as well as part of your entree. Fruits, instead of sweets made with a lot of sugar and fat, are featured for dessert.

Each recipe in this chapter includes a nutritional breakdown per serving. The total calories, protein, fat, carbohydrate, and cholesterol are given. The relative exchange value for each serving is also noted, for those following one of the Sample Weight-Loss Plans discussed in

Chapter 14. In figuring the exchange value for each recipe, the nutrient composition was first determined using standard food composition tables. The relative exchange value for each serving was then calculated from this information. (See Chapter 14 and Appendix A for more information). And, for your convenience, some recipes are noted as "quick," which means that they take less than thirty minutes to prepare.

We recommend the use of whole-wheat pastry flour in all recipes requiring a light texture (cakes, cookies, pancakes, and some breads). The flour should be ground from soft spring wheat. We've found the El Molino brand to work most effectively compared with the other nationally marketed brands.

You may substitute enriched all-purpose flour for whole-wheat pastry flour in these recipes, though the product will not be as nourishing (see Chapter 4 for more information). You may also use regular whole-wheat flour (anything that does not specifically say "pastry flour" on the label), but a somewhat heavier texture will result. If you do this, be sure to sift the flour to remove the larger pieces of bran so the baked product won't turn out too heavy.

Regular whole-wheat bread flour is best for breads, both the knead and the no-knead varieties. It does not have to be sifted for use in these breads, as they can tolerate a heavier texture.

Better Breakfasts

WHOLE-WHEAT AND OAT CEREAL

4 cups water
1 cup whole wheat berries*
1 cup whole oat groats*

EACH SERVING PROVIDES
74 calories
3 g protein
1 g fat
15 g carbohydrate
0 mg cholesterol

OR EXCHANGES AS FOLLOWS
1 bread

Boil water. Add grains and boil for 5 minutes uncovered. Then cover tightly and turn down heat. Simmer for 50 minutes. Turn off heat and leave covered another 15 minutes.

Makes approximately 12 half-cup servings. Can be stored at least one week in the refrigerator.

This cereal and the recipes that follow are good sources of fiber, potassium, magnesium, and other key nutrients.

*Wheat berries and oat groats are the unprocessed seed grains. These are available in natural-food stores.

MUESLI

1/2 cup cooked wheat and oat cereal
6 green grapes
2 tbsp raisins
8 raw almonds, chopped
1/2 small tart apple, diced
1/2 cup lowfat milk

EACH SERVING PROVIDES
350 calories
11 g protein
8 g fat
66 g carbohydrate
6 mg cholesterol

OR EXCHANGES AS FOLLOWS
1/2 milk
2 fruit
2 1/2 bread
1 1/2 fat

Pour fruits, nuts, and milk over cereal. Serve cold. Makes one serving.

A refreshing summer breakfast or light dinner after a hot day. Allow 10 to 15 minutes' chewing time. Great for your jaw muscles and gums.

DATE-NUT CEREAL

1/2 cup cooked wheat and oat
  cereal
1/2 cup lowfat milk
Cinnamon to taste
4 dates, sliced
6 walnut halves, chopped

EACH SERVING PROVIDES
303 calories
11 g protein
8 g fat
53 g carbohydrate
6 mg cholesterol

OR EXCHANGES AS FOLLOWS
1/2 milk
2 fruit
1 1/2 bread
1/2 meat
1 fat

Warm cereal in milk spiced with cinnamon. Best to bring milk to simmer with cereal in it. Then cover and turn off heat. Let cereal sit on hot burner while you prepare the dates and nuts.

Pour dates and nuts over warmed cereal and enjoy. Serves one.

BAKED SWEDISH PANCAKE

2 tbsp butter or margarine
1 1/2 cups lowfat milk
1 cup whole-wheat pastry flour
1 1/2 tbsp sugar
1/4 tsp salt
1/2 tsp ground cardamom
3 eggs
Grated peel of 1 lemon

EACH SERVING PROVIDES
289 calories
13 g protein
13 g fat
33 g carbohydrate
213 mg cholesterol

OR EXCHANGES AS FOLLOWS
1/2 milk
1 1/2 bread

Place the butter in a 2″ × 8″ × 14″ baking dish and melt it in the preheating oven (425°F).

Meanwhile, mix all other ingredients. When the butter has melted, pour the batter into the dish and immediately return dish to oven. (If baking dish cools off, the pancake will not puff up as nicely.) Bake until deep brown and puffy (about 35 minutes). It will be moist inside and crisp on the outside. Serves 4.

Eating this pancake is a memorable treat. Best served with unsweetened berries, fresh peaches, bananas, or

1 meat
2 fat
1 tsp sugar

fresh applesauce. You may want to add just a dab of real maple syrup.

For a baked apple or pear pancake, substitute cinnamon for the cardamom and add 1 sliced tart apple or pear to the batter. Reduce the milk to 1 1/4 cups.

Each serving provides 302 calories, 13 g protein, 12 g fat, 38 g carbohydrate, 213 mg cholesterol. Just figure 1/2 fruit added to exchanges per serving for the original recipe.

BLUEBERRY BREAKFAST CREPES

CREPES
3 eggs
3/4 cup lowfat milk
1 1/2 tsp oil
1/4 tsp salt
3/4 cup whole-wheat pastry
   flour

CHEESE FILLING
1 1/2 cups ricotta cheese
3 tbsp real maple syrup
3/4 tsp vanilla
3/8 tsp cinnamon
2 tsp butter (for baking dish)

BLUEBERRY GARNISH
2 12-oz pkg frozen blueberries
   (no sugar added)
Sifted powdered sugar

To make the crepes, beat eggs, milk, oil and salt together. Add flour a small amount at a time. Beat into a smooth batter. Let sit at room temperature while you make the cheese filling.

To make the cheese filling, beat together all the ingredients listed, except the butter. Use this to grease the baking dish.

To cook the crepes, heat a 7" skillet and coat lightly with oil. For each crepe, pour in 3 tbsp batter. Tilt skillet in several directions to coat it with a thin layer of batter. Turn crepe as soon as surface becomes dull. Fry lightly on the other side. Stack on a plate with wax paper underneath each crepe. The crepes may be frozen at this stage for later use if they are well sealed in freezer wrap.

EACH SERVING PROVIDES
438 calories
21 g protein
17 g fat
54 g carbohydrate
225 mg cholesterol

OR EXCHANGES AS FOLLOWS
1 fruit
2 bread
2 1/2 meat
2 fat
3 tsp sugar

To assemble crepes, fill each with 2 rounded tbsp of cheese filling. Roll up and place in baking dish with the tuck on the bottom and each one touching the other. Cover the dish with foil and heat at 350°F for 20 minutes until warmed thoroughly. While the crepes are warming, prepare the blueberries.

To prepare the blueberries, heat them in a heavy saucepan until just warmed. Try not to overheat, as they will become mushy.

Serves 4 (3 crepes each). Garnish each serving with 1/2 to 2/3 cup of warmed berries. Sift a little powdered sugar on top and serve on warm plates with a sprig of parsley for color.

WHOLE-WHEAT BUTTERMILK PANCAKES

4 eggs
1/4 tsp baking soda
1/4 tsp salt
1 1/2 cups buttermilk
1 cup whole-wheat pastry flour
3 tbsp oil

EACH SERVING PROVIDES
334 calories
15 g protein
19 g fat
29 g carbohydrate
258 mg cholesterol

OR EXCHANGES AS FOLLOWS
1/2 milk
1 1/2 bread
1 meat
3 fat

Separate the yolks from the eggs. Beat the egg yolks, soda, and salt together until frothy. Add the buttermilk, flour, and 2 tbsp of the oil. Mix briefly. It is important that you do not overstir or the pancakes will be tough.

Now beat the egg whites until siff. Fold these into the pancake mixture.

Fry in a skillet lightly oiled as needed with the remaining 1 tbsp of oil. Makes approximately 20 3-inch thin and delicate pancakes. Serves 4.

DARK, MOIST BRAN MUFFINS

1/2 cup raisins, plumped
1 1/2 tbsp orange rind, grated finely
2 cups whole wheat flour
1 1/2 cups unprocessed bran
2 tbsp sugar
1/4 tsp salt
1 1/4 tsp baking soda
1 egg
1/2 cup blackstrap molasses
2 tbsp oil
2 cups buttermilk

EACH MUFFIN PROVIDES
87 calories
3 g protein
2 g fat
16 g carbohydrate
12 mg cholesterol

OR EXCHANGES AS FOLLOWS
1 bread
1/2 fat

Soak raisins in 1/2 cup boiling water until plumped. Drain just before adding to the recipe. Grate orange rind.

Mix in a large bowl the flour, bran, sugar, salt, and soda. Combine the raisins, orange rind, egg, molasses, oil, and buttermilk in a separate bowl. Then add the wet ingredients (all at once) to the dry ingredients. Stir just enough to moisten the flour mixture.

Fill paper-lined muffin tins 2/3 full and bake at 350°F for 20 to 25 minutes. Remove muffins from tin right away to cool on wire racks. This helps to keep them from sticking to the muffin papers. Makes 24 muffins.

These muffins are very moist, light, and delicious. Also a good source of iron and fiber.

Try replacing 1/4 cup of flour with 1/4 cup of soya flour to enhance the protein quality.

DATE BRAN MUFFINS

3 cups All-Bran cereal
8 oz dates, chopped
1 1/3 cups boiling water
1/4 cup butter
1/4 cup safflower oil .
3 eggs
2 cups buttermilk
2 1/2 cups whole wheat pastry flour
1/2 tsp salt
2 tsp soda

Pour boiling water over bran cereal and dates. Let stand while you beat together the butter, oil, and eggs.

Mix the dry ingredients. Add dry ingredients alternately with buttermilk to the date mixture.

Bake in muffin papers in a 400°F oven for 15 minutes.

Makes 36 muffins. Batter will keep in the refrigerator for several weeks.

BLUEBERRY MUFFINS

2 1/4 cups wholewheat flour
1/4 cup unprocessed bran
1/4 tsp salt
1 1/4 tsp baking soda
1 egg
1/3 cup mild honey
1/4 cup oil
1 3/4 cups buttermilk
1 1/2 cups frozen blueberries
  (no sugar added)

Combine the flour, bran, salt and soda. Beat together the egg, honey, oil, and buttermilk. Stir the egg mixture into the flour mixture, just enough to moisten. Then fold in the blueberries.

Fill paper-lined muffin tins 2/3 full and bake at 400°F for 20 minutes or until browned. Remove muffins from tins right away to cool on wire racks. This will help to keep them from sticking to the muffin papers. Makes 20 muffins.

Try substituting 1/4 cup soya flour for 1/4 cup whole-wheat flour to improve the protein quality of these muffins.

BRAN DATE BREAD

1 1/2 cups whole wheat pastry
  flour
1 tbsp baking powder
1 tsp salt

Mix dry ingredients. Blend in all the rest of the ingredients. Do not overstir or the bread will be tough. Bake in a

1 1/2 cups unprocessed bran
1/2 cup chopped dates
1 egg
3/4 cup nonfat milk
1/2 cup real maple syrup
1/4 cup oil

EACH SLICE PROVIDES
115 calories
3 g protein
3 g fat
20 g carbohydrate
16 mg cholesterol

OR EXCHANGES AS FOLLOWS
1/2 fruit
1 bread
1/2 fat

greased loaf pan at 350°F for approximately 50 minutes. Makes 16 slices.

BANANA FRUIT BREAD

1/3 cup butter or margarine
1/3 cup sugar
2 eggs
3 large bananas, mashed
1/4 cup buttermilk
1 1/4 cups whole-wheat pastry
    flour
1 tsp baking powder
1/2 tsp salt
1/2 tsp baking soda
1 cup unprocessed bran
3/4 cup finely diced apricots
1/2 cup chopped walnuts

EACH SLICE PROVIDES
164 calories
4 g protein
7 g fat
25 g carbohydrate
43 mg cholesterol

OR EXCHANGES AS FOLLOWS
1 fruit
1 bread
1 fat

Cream together the butter and sugar. Add eggs and beat well. In a separate bowl, mix the bananas and milk. Set aside. In another bowl, combine the flour, baking powder, salt, soda, bran, dried fruit, and nuts. Now, stir flour mixture into creamed mixture alternately with banana mixture.

Bake in a greased loaf pan at 350°F for 60 minutes or until done. Makes 16 slices.

HIGH-FIBER PUMPKIN BREAD

1/2 cup brown sugar, packed
1/2 cup oil
2 eggs
2 cups canned pumpkin
1 1/2 cups whole-wheat pastry
    flour
1 cup unprocessed bran
1/2 tsp soda
1/4 tsp salt
1/2 tsp cinnamon
1/2 tsp nutmeg
1/4 tsp allspice
1/4 tsp cloves
1/4 tsp baking powder
1 cup raisins
1/2 cup walnuts, chopped

EACH SLICE PROVIDES
192 calories
4 g protein
10 g fat
24 g carbohydrate
31 mg cholesterol

OR EXCHANGES AS FOLLOWS
1/2 fruit.
1 bread
2 fat
2 tsp sugar

Mix sugar, oil, eggs, and pumpkin. Stir together all the rest of the ingredients in a separate bowl. Combine the wet ingredients with the dry ingredients. Be careful not to overstir, as this causes the product to become tough.

Pour into a lightly oiled loaf pan and bake at 350°F for 1 hour. Remove from oven and cool in pan for 20 minutes. Then take out of the pan and cool completely on a wire rack. Makes 16 slices.

Good source of vitamin A and iron, in addition to fiber.

SWEET WHEAT LAMBKINS COFFEE CAKE

DOUGH
2 pkg. active dry yeast
1/2 cup lukewarm water
1/2 cup sugar
2 eggs, lightly beaten
1/2 tsp salt
1/2 cup melted butter
1 tsp grated lemon rind
1/2 cup lowfat milk
1/2 cup hot water

In a small bowl, mix the yeast, warm water and 1 tsp of the sugar. Let stand while you combine the remaining sugar, eggs, salt, melted butter, lemon rind, milk, and hot water in a large bowl. After the yeast has bubbled up, add it to the egg and butter mixture. Then mix in the whole-wheat flour and beat well to make a soft dough. Turn onto a lightly floured board and

3 cups whole-wheat bread flour
  (do not use pastry flour)
1/2 to 1 1/2 cups unbleached
  white flour

FILLING
1/3 cup sugar
1 tsp cinnamon
1 cup raisins
2 tbsp melted butter

EACH ROLL PROVIDES
120 calories
2 g protein
5 g fat
19 g carbohydrate
27 mg cholesterol

OR EXCHANGES AS FOLLOWS
1 bread
1 fat
1 tsp sugar

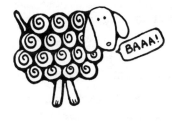

knead until dough is smooth and satiny, about 15 minutes. Flour board and your hands as needed with the unbleached flour.

When dough is smooth and satiny, place it in an oiled bowl and turn it over so the oil also covers the top. Let rise in a warm place until more than doubled in bulk (about 1 1/2 hours). Punch down and divide dough in half.

Cut off a quarter of each half of the dough and reserve to make head, ears, tail and legs of the "lambkins." Roll the remaining dough so that it is about 18″ × 10″. Brush lightly with melted butter. Sprinkle with half of the cinnamon sugar. Then sprinkle with half the raisins. Roll the dough so that you have an 18″ long cylinder. Cut this into 16 equal pieces. Brush edges with a little melted butter and place on a foil-covered cookie sheet as illustration demonstrates.

Now roll the remaining quarter of the dough. Cut a triangle about 4″ on each side for the head. Then cut 2 long ears and 3 long narrow pieces for the tail and legs. Roll a tiny ball of dough for the nose and use two raisins for the eyes.

Repeat for the other half of the dough. Cover each with a tea towel. Let rise in a warm place until doubled in bulk (about 1 hour).

Bake in a preheated 350°F oven for about 20 minutes or until golden brown. Makes 36 rolls.

WALNUT LEMON WHEAT LOAF

2 pkg active dry yeast
1/2 cup lukewarm water
1/4 cup honey
3 tbsp oil
1 tbsp grated lemon peel
2 1/4 cups water
1 cup white flour, unsifted
2 1/4 to 3 1/4 cups whole-wheat
    flour, unsifted
1 1/2 tsp salt
2 cups whole wheat flour,
    unsifted
1 cup chopped walnuts

EACH SLICE PROVIDES
115 calories
3 g protein
4 g fat
18 g carbohydrate
0 mg cholesterol

OR EXCHANGES AS FOLLOWS
1 bread
1 fat

Dissolve the yeast in a lukewarm water. Combine honey, shortening, and lemon peel. Add dissolved yeast and remainder of water to honey mixture. Combine 1 cup white flour and 1 cup whole-wheat flour with the salt, stirring well to blend. Now add flour mixture to yeast mixture. Beat in 1 cup whole-wheat flour until thick and elastic. Stir in remaining 2 cups of whole-wheat flour and the nuts. Then gradually add enough of the remaining flour to make a soft dough that leaves the sides of the bowl.

Turn onto a floured board and round into a ball. Knead 5 to 10 minutes or until the dough is smooth and elastic. Cover and let rise in a warm place free of drafts until doubled in size.

Punch down and shape into two loaves. Place in two greased loaf pans and let rise again until doubled in size.

Bake at 400°F for 30 to 40 minutes. Remove from pans immediately and let cool on wire racks.

Makes 2 loaves, 16 slices per loaf.

Leave out the nuts for a less fattening version: 95 calories, 3 g protein, 2 g fat, 18 g carbohydrate, 0 mg cholesterol per serving.

Entrees—
Meat, Fish,
Poultry

POULET BONNE FEMME

3 to 4 lb roasting chicken
1 large onion, sliced thinly
2 to 3 medium carrots, sliced
  thinly
1 cup dry white wine
1/4 tsp salt
1/8 tsp pepper
1/2 tsp rosemary
1/2 tsp thyme
1 large clove garlic, crushed

EACH SERVING PROVIDES
190 calories
23 g protein
9 g fat
5 g carbohydrate
75 mg cholesterol

OR EXCHANGES AS FOLLOWS
1 vegetable
3 meat

Place chicken in bottom of a large casserole. Add vegetables, wine, and seasonings. Cover tightly and bake at 400°F for 75 minutes or until the chicken is tender.

Remove the juice from the pan. Remove fat from it and then thicken it with 1 to 2 tbs cornstarch (mixed first with a little cool water to avoid lumps).

Serve chicken and vegetables with a baked potato. Pour gravy over top of all these, so that you will need only a minimum of spread on your potato. Best with a fresh and crispy green salad. Serves 6.

WELLSPRING CHICKEN

3 to 4 lb roasting chicken
1 onion, chopped coarsely
3 carrots, halved
2 large cloves garlic, crushed
1/4 tsp ground cumin
1/8 tsp salt
Juice of 1 lemon

EACH PORTION PROVIDES
190 calories
23 g protein

Place chicken in the bottom of a large casserole or roasting pan. Spread onion and carrots around it. Sprinkle the seasoning over the chicken and vegetables.

Cover and roast for 60 minutes at 450°F. Serves 6.

Accompany chicken with roasted veg-

9 g fat
5 g carbohydrate
75 mg cholesterol

etables and a potato or rice, plus a salad.

OR EXCHANGES AS FOLLOWS
1 vegetable
3 meat

TURKEY CREPES WITH VELOUTÉ SAUCE

TURKEY
2 1/2 lbs turkey breast
3 cups hot water
1 onion
5 whole cloves
3 celery tops (leaves)
1 bay leaf
1 carrot

VELOUTÉ SAUCE
3 tbsp turkey or chicken fat
3 tbsp flour
Dash cayenne pepper
1 1/2 cups turkey broth

CREPES
See recipe for crepes under
  Manicotti with Raisins and
  Walnuts in Entrees-
  Vegetarian section

EACH SERVING PROVIDES
403 calories
35 g protein
22 g fat
17 g carbohydrate
223 mg cholesterol

OR EXCHANGES AS FOLLOWS
1 bread
4 1/2 meat
1 1/2 fat

To prepare the turkey, place turkey, water, onion (stuck with cloves), celery leaves, bay leaf, and carrot in a pressure cooker. Cook at 15 pounds pressure for 25 to 35 minutes, or as manufacturer directs. Reduce pressure slowly.

Remove the turkey from the broth as soon as you can remove the lid. Refrigerate until you are ready to use it. Strain the broth and cool it until the fat rises to the top and you can remove it. Reserve the fat for use in the sauce.

2 1/2 pounds of raw turkey breast will yield approximately 7 3-oz portions of cooked meat. Freeze any left over for use later.

To prepare the sauce, melt the fat in a heavy saucepan. Mix in flour and cayenne. Stir in broth and simmer slowly until thickened and smooth. Reserve 1/3 of this sauce to pour over the prepared crepes.

To prepare the turkey filling, cut 12 ounces cooked turkey into bite-size pieces. Add these to the 2/3 of the sauce left in the saucepan. Warm thoroughly over low heat. Be careful not to overheat or overstir, or the turkey will shred.

To assemble the crepes, spoon turkey sauce into heated crepes. Roll up crepe and place seam-side down on warmed plates. Spoon a little of the reserved sauce onto the crepes. Garnish with parsley or watercress. Serves 4.

FISH WITH FINE HERBS

1 lb. halibut (or other firm-
  fleshed fish)
1/2 tsp herb salt
1/8 tsp basil
1/8 tsp marjoram
1/8 tsp chervil or dried parsley
1/2 cup white wine
1 1/2 tbs lemon juice
1 tbsp cornstarch
3/4 cup fresh mushrooms,
  chopped finely
1/2 cup grated cheddar cheese

EACH PORTION PROVIDES
188 calories
29 g protein
6 g fat
3 g carbohydrate
88 mg cholesterol

OR EXCHANGES AS FOLLOWS
3 meats

Place fish filets in a casserole. Mix the salt and herbs into the wine and lemon juice. Pour this combination over the fish and marinate in the refrigerator for at least 30 minutes. Drain off the liquid and thicken slightly over low heat with the cornstarch.

Add the mushrooms and cheese to the thickened sauce. Spread this mixture over the fish. Bake at 400°F for about 25 minutes or until the sauce begins to bubble evenly at the edges. Garnish with minced parsley. Serves 4.

MUSHROOMS STUFFED WITH CRAB

20 very large fresh mushrooms
1/2 lb crab meat, shredded
20 mushroom stems, chopped
  finely
1 cup grated jack cheese
1 egg, lightly beaten

Clean and remove stems from mushrooms. Place mushrooms right side up in a lightly buttered skillet. Add about 1 tbsp water. Cover tightly and cook over low heat until they are

1 tbsp white wine
1/2 tsp herb salt
Dash cayenne pepper
1 cup soft white bread crumbs
1/2 cup white sauce

EACH SERVING PROVIDES
300 calories
24 g protein
17 g fat
14 g carbohydrate
169 mg cholesterol

OR EXCHANGES AS FOLLOWS
1 vegetable
1/2 bread
3 meat
1 1/2 fat

slightly soft to the touch. Then turn them over and turn off the heat.

In the meantime, mix thoroughly the crab, mushroom stems, 1/2 cup cheese, egg, wine, salt, and cayenne. Combine the bread crumbs with the cream sauce. Then mix this into the crab mixture.

Cover each mushroom with a generous scoop of the crab mixture. Sprinkle the remaining 1/2 cup of cheese over the top and bake at 400°F until mushrooms begin to simmer. Serves 4.

HERBED CHICKEN

3 to 4 lb roasting chicken
1/2 tsp dry mustard
1/2 tsp ground marjoram
1/2 tsp ground thyme
3/4 tsp ground sage
4 to 5 bay leaves
Pepper to taste

EACH SERVING PROVIDES
165 calories
21 g protein
9 g fat
0 g carbohydrate
75 mg cholesterol

OR EXCHANGES AS FOLLOWS
3 meat

Place chicken in the bottom of a casserole or roasting pan. Sprinkle with seasonings. Cover and bake at 450°F for 45 minutes. (If you bake two chickens at once, increase the heat to 475°F.)

Turn oven down to 375°F and bake another 10–15 minutes. Serves 6.

ROAST VEAL PRINTEMPS

3 lbs rump veal roast, rolled
2 tbsp butter or margarine
1/4 tsp salt
1/2 tsp pepper
1/2 tsp rosemary
1/2 cup beef consommé
1/2 cup dry white wine
2 tbs flour
1/4 cup water

EACH SERVING PROVIDES
221 calories
22 g protein
13 g fat
1 g carbohydrate
88 mg cholesterol

OR EXCHANGES AS FOLLOWS
3 meat
1 fat

Quickly brown veal in butter. Season with salt, pepper, and rosemary. Place veal in roasting pan and pour consommé and white wine over it. Cover tightly.

Roast in a preheated 400°F oven for 2 hours or until veal is tender. Pour off juices into a skillet. Mix flour and water together and then stir into the gravy. Simmer a few minutes until the gravy thickens.

Slice the veal. Pour gravy over each portion. Serves 12.

CIOPPINO
(Italian Fish Soup)

SAUCE
1/8 cup olive oil
1 tbsp chopped garlic
1/8 cup chopped parsley
1/8 cup chopped celery
1/8 cup chopped green pepper
2 15-oz. cans tomato purée
1/2 tsp salt
1 tbsp paprika
1/2 cup sherry
1 tbsp dry basil
1 cup water

SOUP
4 summer squash, sliced into
    bite-size pieces
2 green peppers, seeded and
    chopped

To prepare the sauce, sauté the first four ingredients in the oil for five minutes. Add all the other ingredients and simmer at low heat for 45 to 60 minutes. (The flavor improves if the sauce is made a day ahead. It's also a good idea to make a double batch and freeze half for later use.)

To prepare the soup, heat the sauce to boiling. Stir in all the vegetables (except the parsley) and the fish. Simmer covered for 10 minutes, until the fish flakes and vegetables are barely tender.

2 cups fresh string beans, cut
  into small pieces
12 medium fresh mushrooms,
  sliced
2/3 cup chopped parsley
1 lb firm-fleshed white fish, cut
  into bite-size pieces

Serve in large bowls garnished with
the parsley. Great with crusty bread.
Serves 4.

EACH SERVING PROVIDES
391 calories
34 g protein
9 g fat
40 g carbohydrate
75 mg cholesterol

OR EXCHANGES AS FOLLOWS
8 vegetable
3 meat

POACHED FISH (QUICK)

1 lb firm-fleshed fish
1 cup chicken broth
1 medium onion, chopped finely
2 cups sliced mushrooms
1/4 tsp herb salt
1 1/2 tbsp butter or margarine

Simmer the onion in the broth for 5
minutes, uncovered. Add fish, mushrooms and salt. Cover and simmer an
additional 10 minutes. Remove from
heat and drain liquid into a small
saucepan. Thicken over heat by adding 1 to 2 tbsp cornstarch (mixed first
in a small amount of cool liquid to
avoid lumps). Swirl in butter or margarine.

EACH SERVING PROVIDES
174 calories
25 g protein
5 g fat
6 g carbohydrate
89 mg cholesterol

OR EXCHANGES AS FOLLOWS
1 vegetable
3 meat

Serve sauce over fish. Garnish with
chopped parsley. Accompany with
rice or a baked potato, plus a steamed
vegetable and a salad. Serves 4.

POACHED FISH WITH HORSERADISH SAUCE (QUICK)

1 1/2 lbs fish fillets about 1"
   thick
3/4 cup chicken broth
4 oz neufchatel cheese (lowfat
   cream cheese)
1 tbsp prepared horseradish
1 tbsp butter or margarine
2 tbsp flour
Salt and pepper to taste
Chopped green onion or parsley
   for garnish

EACH SERVING PROVIDES
254 calories
32 g protein
11 g fat
4 g carbohydrate
142 mg cholesterol

OR EXCHANGES AS FOLLOWS
4 1/2 meat

Arrange fish in a 10-inch frying pan. Pour chicken broth over it. Cover and simmer just until fish flakes easily when tested with a fork at the thickest part, about 20 minutes.

Lift fish out of pan with a slotted spoon and arrange on a serving dish. Keep warm. Measure cooking broth; you should have about 1 cup. If you have more, boil it to reduce; if less, add broth to make 1 cup.

Meanwhile, combine neufchatel cheese, horseradish, and 1/3 cup of the cooking broth. Stir until smooth and set aside.

In the frying pan, melt butter over medium heat. Add flour and cook until bubbly. Remove from heat and stir in the remaining 2/3 cup cooking broth until smooth. Cook, stirring constantly, until sauce boils and thickens. Continue to stir constantly with wire whisk and gradually add hot sauce to cheese mixture. Return sauce to pan, adding any juices accumulated on fish plate. Cook, stirring, until it boils. Add salt and pepper to taste.

Pour sauce over fish. Garnish with finely chopped green onion or parsley. Makes 4 servings.

Entrees—Vegetarian

MUSHROOM STROGANOFF (QUICK)

14 oz noodles or spaghetti
2 bay leaves
Garlic powder to taste
Scant salt and pepper
2 medium onions, chopped
4 tsp oil
1 1/4 lbs fresh mushrooms,
  sliced
2 cloves garlic
Dash ground cloves
2 vegetable bouillon cubes
1/4 cup water
1/4 cup sherry
1 tbsp cornstarch
8 oz sour cream
1/4 cup parsley, minced

EACH SERVING PROVIDES
617 calories
19 g protein
18 g fat
89 g carbohydrate
32 mg cholesterol

OR EXCHANGES AS FOLLOWS
3 vegetable
5 bread
1/2 meat
3 1/2 fat

Bring large pot of water to a boil. Add bay leaves and noodles and boil uncovered for 10 minutes. Drain noodles, remove bay leaves and put noodles back into cooking pot. Now add 1 tsp oil, garlic powder, salt, and pepper. Toss seasoning through noodles. (The oil will keep the noodles from sticking together.) Cover and keep warm until serving time.

Meanwhile, sauté the onions in 3 tsp oil until lightly browned. Add the sliced mushrooms, garlic, and cloves. Cover and simmer until the mushrooms soften. While mushrooms are cooking, mix the bouillon cubes, water, sherry, and cornstarch. When the mushrooms are tender, add the bouillon mixture and simmer until thickened. Stir in the sour cream. Warm through, being careful that the sour cream does not get too hot, because it will curdle.

Serve stroganoff over noodles. Garnish with generous amount of minced parsley. Best with a steamed vegetable and crisp salad. Men love this dish! Serves 4.

EGGPLANT AND TOMATO CASSEROLE

1/4 cup olive oil
1 medium onion, chopped
3/4 lb fresh mushrooms, sliced
1/2 medium green pepper,
    sliced
1 medium eggplant, cut into 1"
    cubes
1 15-oz can tomato sauce
1/4 cup parsley, minced
1 cup Parmesan cheese, grated
1 cup mozzarella cheese, grated
2 eggs, beaten
1/3 cup raw sunflower seeds

EACH SERVING PROVIDES
382 calories
16 g protein
23 g fat
20 g carbohydrate
103 mg cholesterol

OR EXCHANGES AS FOLLOWS
1 1/2 bread
2 meat
3 1/2 fat

Sauté mushrooms and onions over medium heat until tender. Stir in green pepper, eggplant, tomato sauce, and parsley. Cover and simmer slowly until eggplant is tender (about 20 minutes), stirring often to prevent sticking. If you need to reduce liquid, uncover and increase heat briefly.

Meanwhile, combine cheeses with eggs. Spoon half eggplant mixture into a 2 1/2-quart casserole. Top with half cheese mixture. Repeat layers ending with cheese. Sprinkle sunflower seeds on top. Bake uncovered in a 375°F oven for 25 minutes. Serves 6.

Accompany with pasta or crusty bread and a mixed vegetable salad.

BUBBLE AND SQUEAK (QUICK)

4 cups cooked brown rice
4 medium summer squash (use
    a variety of zucchini, crook-
    neck, and patty-pan), cubed
3 cups tomato sauce (preferably
    homemade; see Dips, Spreads,
    Sauces section)
1 cup grated cheddar cheese

EACH SERVING PROVIDES
545 calories
20 g protein
21 g fat

Warm up rice in a steamer over boiling water. Steam squash until barely tender (should remain slightly crunchy so it "squeaks" when eaten). Warm up tomato sauce. Divide rice among 4 oven-proof plates. Spoon squash over rice. Cover with tomato sauce. Top with cheese. Put under broiler briefly until cheese melts and tomato sauce bubbles. Serves 4.

72 g carbohydrate
30 mg cholesterol

OR EXCHANGES AS FOLLOWS
2 vegetable
4 bread
1 meat
3 1/2 fat

You may wish to garnish each serving with some minced parsley for added color. Serve with a tossed green salad.

CARROT AND MUSHROOM BAKE WITH ASPARAGUS SAUCE

1 tbsp olive oil
1 lb young carrots, chopped
   finely
1/4 lb fresh mushrooms,
   minced
1/4 medium onion, chopped
   finely
1 cup fat-free stock (vegetable
   or chicken)
1/8 tsp salt
1/8 tsp pepper
2 eggs, beaten lightly
3 oz cheddar or jack cheese,
   grated (about 3/4 cup)
1/4 tsp chervil (optional)
1/4 cup fresh parsley, minced
3/4 lb fresh green asparagus (or
   1 pkg frozen)
1/2 cup vegetable or chicken
   stock
2 tbsp sour cream

EACH SERVING PROVIDES
253 calories
14 g protein
15 g fat
16 g carbohydrate
144 mg cholesterol

OR EXCHANGES AS FOLLOWS
1 bread
1 1/2 meat
2 fat

Sauté carrots, mushrooms, and onion in oil for about 3 minutes. Add stock, salt, and pepper. Cover and cook for 5 minutes. Uncover and cook over moderate heat for 5 to 10 more minutes. Liquid should be evaporated but carrots should not be dry.

Meanwhile, combine lightly beaten eggs, cheese, chervil, and parsley. Add sautéed vegetables to egg mixture. Pour into a buttered 1-pint ring mold or 9″ square Pyrex pan. Cover and place in hot water. Bake at 425°F for 25 to 30 minutes (or until mixture is completely set).

While the carrot mixture is baking, cut the asparagus into 1″ pieces after snapping off tough lower portion of stem. Cook asparagus in a minimum of water until barely tender. Combine cooked asparagus with 1/4 cup cooking liquid, 1/2 cup stock, and sour cream in blender container. Purée.

Unmold carrot mixture onto platter (or cut into serving pieces and place onto plates). Pour asparagus purée around it or over top. Decorate center with sprigs of parsley. Serves 4.

Based on a recipe from *Cuisine Minceur* (see Suggested Reading List in Appendix C).

SPAGHETTI WITH CAULIFLOWER SAUCE (QUICK)

1 lb spaghetti
1/8 cup olive oil
1 lb (1 medium) cauliflower,
   broken into 1" flowerets
3 medium cloves garlic, minced
1 bay leaf, broken into several
   pieces
2 tsp dried basil
2 cups tomato purée
Salt and pepper
1 1/2 cups grated cheddar
   cheese

EACH SERVING PROVIDES
527 calories
22 g protein
19 g fat
67 g carbohydrate
40 mg cholesterol

OR EXCHANGES AS FOLLOWS
1 vegetable
4 bread
2 meat
2 1/2 fat

Boil spaghetti in water until barely tender. Drain and toss with 1/2 tbsp of the olive oil. Salt and pepper to taste.

Meanwhile, sauté the cauliflower in 1 1/2 tbsp of the olive oil for about 3 to 5 minutes. Add the garlic, bay leaf, basil, and tomato purée. Simmer covered for 15 minutes.

Meanwhile, grate the cheese.

Serve cauliflower sauce over the spaghetti and top with the cheese.

Makes 6 servings.

SPAGHETTI WITH BASIL SAUCE (QUICK)

1/4 cup olive oil
2 tbsp dried basil
1/2 cup fresh parsley, minced
8 cloves garlic, minced
12 oz spaghetti noodles
1 cup Parmesan cheese, grated

EACH SERVING PROVIDES
521 calories
18 g protein
21 g fat
65 g carbohydrate
15 mg cholesterol

OR EXCHANGES AS FOLLOWS
1 vegetable
4 bread
1 meat
3 1/2 fat

Sauté basil, parsley, and garlic in oil until garlic is barely golden. Cook spaghetti until just tender in unsalted water. Toss basil sauce through the spaghetti. Then toss Parmesan cheese through spaghetti. Serves 4.

Accompany with a mixed vegetable salad.

DUTCH PANCAKE WITH SPRING VEGETABLES (QUICK)

PANCAKE
2 eggs
1/2 cup whole-wheat pastry
    flour
1/2 cup lowfat milk
1/4 tsp salt
1 tbsp butter

FILLING
1 lb fresh mushrooms,
    quartered
1/3 lb carrots, cut diagonally
    into 1/4" slices
1 medium zucchini, cut
    diagonally into 1/4" slices
1 tbsp safflower oil
1/2 cup (6 to 7 large) pimento-
    stuffed green olives, sliced
1/2 tsp dried dillweed
1 tsp dried summer savory
1/4 tsp salt

Heat oven to 425°F. Prepare vegetables and grate cheese. Heat a 9" heavy ovenproof skillet in oven until very hot. Meanwhile, mix eggs, flour, milk, and salt. Beat until smooth, about 3 minutes. Remove skillet from oven and add butter. Rotate until butter melts and coats the pan. Add batter and return to oven immediately. If skillet cools off, the pancake will not rise nicely. Bake on lowest oven shelf for 10 minutes. Reduce heat to 350°F. Bake until golden, about another 10 minutes. Remove from oven.

Meanwhile, sauté mushrooms, carrots, and zucchini in oil in a large skillet until liquid evaporates, about 5

1 cup (4 oz) Gouda cheese,
    grated

TOPPING
1/2 cup (2 oz) Gouda cheese,
    grated

EACH SERVING PROVIDES
360 calories
20 g protein
22 g fat
24 g carbohydrate
202 mg cholesterol

OR EXCHANGES AS FOLLOWS
2 vegetable
1 bread
2 meat
3 fat

minutes. If liquid remains, drain it off. Add olives, dill, savory, and salt. Reduce heat to medium-low and stir in cheese. Cook, stirring constantly, until cheese melts and coats vegetables, about 2 minutes.

Heat oven to 550°F and/or broil. Spoon vegetable mixture into pancake and top with 1/2 cup cheese. Broil until light brown (2 minutes or less). Cut into wedges and serve immediately.

Makes 4 servings.

MANICOTTI WITH RAISINS AND WALNUTS*

MANICOTTI CREPES
4 eggs
1 cup lowfat milk
1 cup whole-wheat pastry flour
1 tsp oil

RED SAUCE
2 tbsp olive oil
2 medium onions, chopped
1 medium carrot, chopped
3 large cloves garlic, minced
2 15-oz cans tomato purée
1 8-oz can tomato sauce
1/2 tsp celery seeds (optional)
1/8 tsp black pepper
1/2 tsp salt
1/4 tsp chili powder
1/3 cup fresh parsley, chopped
1 tsp basil
1/4 tsp thyme
1/2 tsp allspice
1/3 cup red wine
1/2 lb mushrooms, chopped

To make crepes, beat eggs, milk, flour, and oil into a smooth batter, adding flour a small amount at a time. Let sit at room temperature while you make red sauce.

To make red sauce, heat olive oil in a large, heavy frying pan. Add chopped onions, carrots, and garlic. Sauté until onions become transparent. Then add tomato sauce, celery seeds, pepper, salt, chili, parsley, basil, thyme, allspice, wine, and mushrooms. Simmer while you make filling and cook crepes.

To make filling, mix ricotta and mozzarella cheeses thoroughly in a large bowl. Stir in salt, egg, nutmeg, walnuts, and raisins. Refrigerate while frying crepes.

2 cups ricotta cheese
1 cup mozzarella cheese, grated
1/8 tsp salt
1 egg, beaten
1/8 tsp nutmeg
1/2 cup walnuts, chopped
1/2 cup raisins
3/4 cup Parmesan cheese,
  grated
  (reserve for topping)

EACH SERVING PROVIDES
480 calories
25 g protein
23 g fat
44 g carbohydrate
203 mg cholesterol

OR EXCHANGES AS FOLLOWS
3 bread
2 1/2 meat
3 fat

To fry crepes, heat a 7" frying pan and coat lightly with oil. For each crepe, pour in 3 tbsp batter. Tilt pan in several directions to coat pan with a thin layer of batter. Turn crepe as soon as surface becomes dull. Fry lightly on other side. Stack on a plate with wax paper underneath each one. (These may be frozen for later use if they are well-sealed in freezer wrap.) Makes approximately 16 manicotti crepes.

To assemble manicotti crepes, pour 1/3 of red sauce in bottom of a lightly oiled 3" × 9" × 13" pan. Fill crepes with cheese filling and roll up. Line up in pan with tuck on bottom (each one touching another). Pour rest of sauce over top. Sprinkle with parmesan cheese. Bake at 350°F for 25 to 30 minutes. Serves 8.

Serve with crusty rolls and a big salad. You can make a double batch, as the crepes freeze well.

*Based on a recipe from *Ritual of the Hearth* by Roberta Stickler.

MANICOTTI STUFFED WITH SPINACH AND CHEESE

1 1/2 tbsp olive oil
1 1/2 cups chopped onions
2 cloves garlic, minced
1/4 tsp rosemary
1/2 tsp thyme
1 tsp oregano
1 tsp basil
1 29-oz can tomato purée
1 6-oz can tomato paste
12 oz manicotti noodles

Sauté onions and garlic in oil until onions become transparent. Stir in herbs, tomato purée, and paste. Simmer over low heat while preparing manicotti (at least 30 minutes).

Cook manicotti a few at a time in a large amount of boiling water, following package directions (usually for

8 oz ricotta cheese
8 oz lowfat cottage cheese
1/2 cup parmesan cheese,
    grated
2 10-oz pkg frozen chopped
    spinach, thawed and well-
    drained
2 eggs
1 cup mozzarella cheese, grated

EACH SERVING PROVIDES
541 calories
35 g protein
15 g fat
68 g carbohydrate
118 mg cholesterol

OR EXCHANGES AS FOLLOWS
1 vegetable
4 bread
2 1/2 meat
1 fat

only 4 minutes). Lift out with slotted spoon and place in bowl of cold water. Combine ricotta, cottage, and parmesan cheeses with spinach and eggs. Blend well. Drain manicotti on paper towels and fill with cheese mixture.

Pour half of the tomato sauce into a 2″ × 9″ × 13″ baking dish. Arrange filled manicotti on top. Pour remaining sauce over them. Cover with foil and bake at 350°F for 40 minutes. Uncover, sprinkle with mozzarella cheese and bake 5 minutes longer. Let stand 5 minutes before serving. Serves 6.

Serve with crusty bread and a tossed green salad.

International
Bean Cookery

Beans are an excellent source of protein, fiber, B-complex vitamins, and vitamin E, as well as additional magnesium and potassium. These recipes are generally low in fat and contain very little cholesterol.

One pound of dried beans, such as Navy, pinto, red, or pink, equals about 2 1/2 cups and yields 5 to 6 cups when cooked.

To prepare the beans, use 3 cups of water for each cup of dry beans. Soak the beans in the cold water overnight or use the quick soak method by bringing the beans and water to a boil, simmering for 2 minutes and then covering and letting stand for 1 hour. (We prefer to soak beans overnight as they seem to be easier to digest.) Drain beans and fill pot with fresh water. (This seems to decrease gas production.) Simmer the beans gently for 1 to 1 1/2 hours or until tender.

Cook a large batch and freeze leftovers. The 16-ounce soft plastic containers in which you buy ricotta cheese and peanut butter work well for storing extra beans and grains.

RANCH-STYLE BEANS WITH SPAGHETTI (QUICK)

12 oz spaghetti
1 bay leaf
2 medium onions, chopped
1 green pepper, chopped
4 tsp oil
2 15-oz cans Ranch-Style beans
Garlic powder to taste
1/3 cup parsley, chopped

EACH SERVING PROVIDES
630 calories
27 g protein
12 g fat
111 g carbohydrate
0 mg cholesterol

Put water for spaghetti on to boil. Add bay leaf for flavor. Meanwhile, chop onions, green pepper, and parsley. Sauté onions and green pepper in 3 tsp oil until onions become transparent. Cook spaghetti. Add beans to sautéed vegetables and simmer together briefly while spaghetti is cooking. When spaghetti is barely tender, drain and then toss spaghetti with 1 tsp oil and garlic powder to taste.

Serve beans over spaghetti. Top with a generous sprinkling of parsley. Accompany with a mixed vegetable salad. Serves 4.

CHILI CON ELOTE (Beans with Corn)

3 tbsp olive oil
1 medium onion, chopped
1 large clove garlic (or 3 small ones), minced
1 medium green pepper, diced
1 cup vegetable stock
1/4 cup tomato paste
2 cups fresh corn (or 1 10-oz pkg frozen)
4 cups cooked kidney or pinto beans (or 2 15-oz cans)
1/2 tsp chili powder
1/2 tsp cumin powder
1 tsp salt (omit if canned beans are used)
1 tsp oregano

Sauté onion in oil until transparent. Add garlic and green pepper. Sauté another 2 to 3 minutes. Add stock, tomato paste, and corn. Mash 2 cups of the beans and add to pot along with whole beans and seasonings. Simmer 30 minutes on low heat. If too watery, remove cover and cook another 10 minutes. Serve with fresh tortillas or rice and a salad. Serves 4.

Based on recipe from *Laurel's Kitchen*. See Suggested Reading List in Appendix C.

EACH SERVING PROVIDES
483 calories
24 g protein
13 g fat
73 g carbohydrate
0 mg cholesterol

OR EXCHANGES AS FOLLOWS
2 vegetable
4 bread
1 1/2 meat
1 1/2 fat

CREAMED BEANS FRANÇAIS

4 cups cooked white beans
  (Great Northern)
1 medium onion, chopped finely
1 large carrot, chopped finely
3 tbsp butter or margarine
2 tbsp flour
1 1/4 cups lowfat milk
1/2 tsp salt
1/3 cup parsley, chopped finely
1/2 cup Parmesan cheese

EACH SERVING PROVIDES
431 calories
23 g protein
14 g fat
55 g carbohydrate
19 mg cholesterol

OR EXCHANGE AS FOLLOWS
2 vegetable
3 bread
2 meat
1 1/2 fat

Sauté onions and carrots in 1 1/2 tbsp butter until tender. Meanwhile, make cream sauce by melting the remaining 1 1/2 tbsp butter in a heavy saucepan. Stir in flour. Gradually add milk, stirring constantly with a wire whisk until sauce thickens. Stir in salt and parsley.

Combine beans, vegetables, and cream sauce in a casserole. Top with cheese. Cover and bake for 45 minutes at 300°F. Serves 4.

Serve with a large vegetable salad. Also great cold in a sandwich with plenty of lettuce and perhaps a thin slice of cheese for added flavor.

SPANISH LIMA BEANS (Quick*)

1 lb (2 1/2 cups) dry lima
  beans*
Water
1/2 tsp salt
2 cloves garlic, minced
1 1/2 tbsp olive oil
1 cup onion, chopped
1 cup green pepper, chopped
1 cup celery, chopped
1 tbsp cornstarch
1 tbsp chili powder
1 cup pitted black olives,
  drained
1 1/2 cups jack cheese, grated

EACH SERVING PROVIDES
468 calories
24 g protein

Soak beans overnight in about 1 quart of water. Cook beans, adding more water as needed to keep covered, for about one hour or until tender. Drain beans and reserve 1/4 cup of liquid. Add salt and garlic. Set aside.

Meanwhile, heat oil in skillet and sauté onions, green pepper, and celery until barely tender but still crunchy. In a 2-quart casserole, combine the cornstarch, chili powder, and remaining bean liquid. Add the beans, sautéed vegetables, olives, and half of the cheese. Mix. Sprinkle with remaining

19 g fat
52 g carbohydrate
30 mg cholesterol

cheese. Cover and bake in a 375°F oven for 20 to 30 minutes.

Makes 6 servings. Nice with a little brown rice and a tossed vegetable salad.

*To save time, the beans can be prepared the evening before you make the dish. Or you can substitute 4 pkg frozen lima beans for the cooked dry beans. Just be sure to boil the frozen beans until tender before combining them with the other casserole ingredients.

PUERTO RICAN GARBANZO BEANS

2 tbsp olive oil
2 medium onions, minced
3 large cloves garlic, minced
1/2 tsp oregano
1/2 tsp basil
1/4 tsp salt
1 cup parsley, minced
1 cup tomato purée
1 medium bell pepper, chopped
2 cups banana squash, grated
   coarsely (do not pack into cup)
2 cups fresh spinach or Swiss
   chard, shredded
2 15-oz cans garbanzo beans,
   drained (save liquid)

Sauté onion in oil until transparent. Add garlic, oregano, basil, and salt. Roll oregano and basil in your hand to release flavor. Sauté for one minute. Add rest of ingredients and simmer covered for 15 minutes (no longer or it will become mushy and lose color and texture). If mixture becomes too dry, add some of reserved bean juice. Serves 4.

Serve over steamed brown rice (Spanish-style, if you have the time to prepare) and with a salad.

EACH SERVING PROVIDES
500 calories
26 g protein
12 g fat
83 g carbohydrate
0 mg cholesterol

MIDDLE EASTERN LENTILS AND RICE

1 large onion, sliced thinly
1/4 cup olive oil
1 cup lentils
3 1/2 cups water, boiling
1 tsp salt
1/2 cup long-grain brown rice

EACH SERVING PROVIDES
392 calories
15 g protein
15 g fat
51 g carbohydrate
0 mg cholesterol

OR EXCHANGES AS FOLLOWS
1 vegetable
3 bread
1 meat
2 1/2 fat

Sauté onion in oil until well browned. This gives extra flavor to the dish. Add lentils, water, salt, and rice to onions. Cover and simmer (without stirring) until lentils and rice are tender. This will take about 40 minutes. The water should evaporate. Serves 4.

Accompany with a mixed vegetable salad and some unflavored lowfat yogurt. Leftovers are delicious served cold with yogurt.

Grains and Vegetables

NEVER-FAIL BROWN RICE

1 lb long-grain brown rice
  (2 1/2 cups raw)
4 1/2 cups water
1 bay leaf (optional)

EACH SERVING PROVIDES
232 calories
5 g protein
2 g fat
50 g carbohydrate
0 mg cholesterol

OR EXCHANGES AS FOLLOWS
3 bread

Bring water to a boil in a heavy sauce-pan with a tight-fitting lid. Add the rice and bay leaf. Continue to boil for 5 minutes uncovered. Then turn heat down to simmer, cover, and cook for another 40 minutes. Turn off burner and let rice sit covered for at least 10 more minutes. It is important that you do not remove the lid on the cooking pan during this entire process. If you do, the rice will get sticky. Makes approximately 8 1-cup servings.

We've specified long-grain brown rice because it does not get sticky as short-grain brown rice often does. We've also suggested that you cook up the whole pound at once. This will save money and energy—both your's and the world's. Store the leftover rice in one-cup portions in your freezer for a quick meal some other time. The frozen rice can be popped out of the plastic storage containers into a steamer basket and warmed over boiling water. This takes about 15 minutes.

ARROZ A LA JARDINERA

3/4 cup chopped onion
  (1 medium)
1 lb zucchini, thinly sliced
2 tbsp butter or margarine
1 cup frozen corn
1 cup canned tomatoes, drained
  and chopped
3 cups cooked brown rice
1/4 tsp oregano
1/4 tsp salt
1/8 tsp pepper

Cook onion and zucchini in butter until barely tender. Add corn, tomatoes, rice, and seasonings. Cover and simmer 10 minutes to warm through. Serves 4.

EACH SERVING PROVIDES
219 calories
5 g protein
8 g fat
37 g carbohydrate
17 mg cholesterol

OR EXCHANGES AS FOLLOWS
1 vegetable
2 bread
1 1/2 fat

BULGUR WHEAT PILAF

1 small carrot, diced
1 medium stalk celery, diced
1/2 green pepper, diced
1/3 cup mushrooms, diced
2 green onions, sliced thinly
1 bay leaf
1 1/2 tbsp oil
1 3/4 cups vegetable stock or
  water
1 cup raw bulgur wheat
1/2 tsp salt

EACH SERVING PROVIDES
217 calories
6 g protein
6 g fat

Prepare the vegetables. Include the celery leaves (a few add a nice flavor; too many may make the dish bitter). Place the oil in a heavy pot with a close-fitting lid. Add all the vegetables and the bay leaf. Stir over medium heat for several minutes. Pour in the stock, bring to a boil, cover and simmer for 5 minutes.

Add the wheat and salt. Bring back to a fast boil. Cook covered over very low heat for 15 minutes. If too moist, uncover and simmer another few min-

37 g carbohydrate
0 mg cholesterol

OR EXCHANGES AS FOLLOWS
1 vegetable
2 bread
1 fat

utes until the liquid evaporates. Serves 4.

See *Laurel's Kitchen* (refer to Suggested Reading List in Appendix C).

PIQUANT VEGETABLE MÉLANGE (QUICK)

2 tbsp safflower or soy oil
1 tbsp cider vinegar
1 tbsp Worcestershire sauce
3/4 tsp sugar
1/8 tsp powdered oregano
1/4 tsp dry mustard
1/2 lb fresh green beans, cut
    into 2" pieces
1/2 lb fresh mushrooms, halved
2 medium zucchini, sliced
2 medium tomatoes, cut into
    wedges

EACH SERVING PROVIDES
129 calories
4 g protein
7 g fat
14 g carbohydrate
0 mg cholesterol

OR EXCHANGES AS FOLLOWS
2 1/2 vegetable
1 1/2 fat

Combine oil, vinegar, Worcestershire, sugar, oregano, and mustard together in a heavy skillet. Bring to a boil and add beans and mushrooms. Return to boiling point, reduce heat, cover and simmer 5 minutes. Add zucchini. Cover and simmer 3 minutes longer. Add tomatoes. Cover and simmer 1 minute.

Serve immediately. If you would rather serve the vegetables chilled, do not cook tomatoes. Cover and refrigerate, adding tomatoes just before serving.

Makes 4 servings

BROCCOLI WITH ORANGE SAUCE (QUICK)

1 cup water
2 lbs broccoli, broken into
    flowerets
1 tbsp olive oil
1 tbsp butter
1/2 cup scallions, minced
2 large garlic cloves, minced
3/4 cup orange juice

Bring water to a boil in a heavy covered saucepan. Add broccoli to rapidly boiling water, return to a boil, cover and cook over medium heat until barely tender.

Drain cooking water into a mug and either drink along with dinner or re-

1/2 cup dry white wine
1 tbsp grated orange rind
1/2 tbsp cornstarch

EACH SERVING PROVIDES
182 calories
9 g protein
7 g fat
22 g carbohydrate
3 mg cholesterol

OR EXCHANGES AS FOLLOWS
1 1/2 bread
1 meat
1 fat

serve in freezer until you have enough to make a soup stock.

Keep broccoli warm in covered saucepan while you complete sauce. That's why it's important to undercook broccoli. If you do not, while it sits it will turn olive green and lose part of its flavor.

While broccoli is cooking, sauté scallions and garlic in the butter and oil for 1 to 2 minutes. Add 3/4 cup of the orange juice, wine, and orange rind. Cook over low heat until reduced slightly. Mix cornstarch with the remaining 1/4 cup of orange juice to soften. Stir into sauce to thicken slightly.

Serve broccoli and spoon sauce over it. Makes 4 servings.

CARROTS AND TURNIPS (QUICK)

1 cup water
1 lb (3 large) fresh carrots
1 lb (3 medium) fresh turnips
1 tbsp butter
Salt and pepper to taste

EACH SERVING PROVIDES
95 calories
4 g protein
3 g fat
15 g carbohydrate
8 mg cholesterol

OR EXCHANGES AS FOLLOWS
2 vegetable
1/2 fat

Bring water to a boil in a heavy covered saucepan. Meanwhile, scrub, peel, and dice carrots and turnips.

Add vegetables to rapidly boiling water, return to a boil, cover and cook over medium heat until tender (between 5 and 10 minutes).

Drain cooking water into a mug and either drink along with dinner or reserve in freezer until you have enough to make a soup stock.

Add butter, salt and pepper to vegetables. Cover and put back on medium heat for a minute to melt butter. Shake pot to distribute butter and seasonings.

Mash with a fork or potato masher and serve immediately.

Serves 4.

GREEN BEAN CRUNCH (QUICK)

1 cup water
1 small onion, cut into quarters
1 large clove garlic, minced
2 1/2 lbs fresh green beans, washed and cut into 1 1/2" pieces
1 tbsp soy sauce
1 tbsp safflower or soy oil
1 tbsp toasted sesame seeds (optional)

EACH SERVING PROVIDES
116 calories
6 g protein
3 g fat
22 g carbohydrate
0 mg cholesterol

OR EXCHANGES AS FOLLOWS
1 1/2 vegetable
1 bread
1 1/2 fat

Bring water to boil in a heavy covered saucepan with onion and garlic. Meanwhile, prepare the beans.

Add beans to boiling water, return to a boil, cover and cook over medium heat until tender-crisp (between 5 and 10 minutes).

Drain cooking water into a mug and either drink along with dinner or reserve in freezer until you have enough to make a soup stock.

Add the oil, soy sauce, and sesame seeds to the beans, tossing gently to distribute.

Serve immediately. Serves 4.

STIR-FRY VEGETABLE MEDLEY (QUICK)

1/2 lb fresh broccoli
1/2 lb fresh asparagus
1/2 lb fresh celery
1 small onion
2 tbsp safflower or soy oil
1/4 tsp salt

About 20 minutes before serving, cut the broccoli into small flowerets. Then cut the asparagus and celery diagonally into 3" pieces. Slice the onion thinly.

Heat the oil in a skillet or wok. Put the onion in first, then add the rest of

EACH SERVING PROVIDES
115 calories
4 g protein
8 g fat
11 g carbohydrate
0 mg cholesterol

OR EXCHANGES AS FOLLOWS
2 vegetable
1 1/2 fat

the vegetables. Stir-fry over high heat until crisp-tender. This will take about 10 minutes. Salt just before serving.

Serves 4. These vegetables are particularly nice with baked chicken or fish.

GARDEN VEGETABLE CHOWDER

2 tbsp safflower oil
1 tbsp butter
2 cups onions, chopped
4 large cloves garlic, minced
3 cups celery, chopped
3 cups carrots, chopped
4 cups potatoes, cubed
1/2 tsp salt
1/2 tsp thyme
1/8 tsp oregano
1/2 tsp celery seed (optional)
1 29-oz can tomato puree
1 1/2 cups water
1 large green pepper, chopped
2 10-oz pkg. frozen corn
1 1/2 tsp Chili Paste with
   Garlic* (optional but great)

Sauté onions in oil and butter until transparent. Add garlic, celery, carrots, potatoes, salt, thyme, oregano, and celery seeds. Sauté another 10 minutes, watching to make sure that potatoes don't stick. Add tomato purée, water, green pepper, and corn. Bring mixture to a boil over medium heat. Cover and simmer 30 minutes or until vegetables are tender. Serves 4.

Serve in large soup bowls, accompanied with whole-grain bread and a salad. It would be a good idea to serve the chowder with some cheese or have a yogurt or custard dessert in order to complement the vegetable protein.

*Chili Paste with Garlic is a condiment available in the Oriental section of the supermarket.

EACH SERVING PROVIDES
437 calories
13 g protein
12 g fat
81 g carbohydrate
9 mg cholesterol

OR EXCHANGES AS FOLLOWS
1 vegetable
5 bread
2 fat

CHILLED LIMA BEAN SOUP (QUICK)

3 cups tomato juice
2 pkg frozen lima beans
1/2 cup parsley, chopped
1/2 green pepper, seeded
2 green onions, sliced
1 cup plain lowfat yogurt
1/4 cup sour cream
1/2 tsp curry powder
Salt and pepper to taste

EACH SERVING PROVIDES
292 calories
14 g protein
6 g fat
47 g carbohydrate
12 mg cholesterol

OR EXCHANGES AS FOLLOWS
3 bread
1 meat
1/2 fat

Keep tomato juice, yogurt and sour cream in refrigerator until ready to use. Do not defrost lima beans.

Prepare the fresh vegetables. Break frozen lima beans into chunks. Put tomato juice, lima beans, and vegetables into a blender and blend until almost smooth. Then add the yogurt, sour cream, curry, salt, and pepper and blend to a smooth purée.

Serve at once garnished with minced parsley or chives and a sprinkle of paprika. Add fresh bread or rolls and a large mixed vegetable salad and you have a quick and refreshing dinner for a warm day.

Serves 4.

Salads

SALAD SAN DIEGO (QUICK)

1 clove garlic
2 cups romaine lettuce, torn
   into pieces
2 cups iceberg lettuce, torn into
   pieces
2 cups red leaf lettuce, torn into
   pieces
1 cup fresh broccoli, broken
   into flowerets and chopped
1 fresh cauliflower, broken into
   flowerets and chopped
2 green onions, sliced thinly
1/2 cup parsley, minced
2 medium tomatoes, cut into
   chunks
2 tbsp olive oil
1/2 tsp dried basil
Pinch dried thyme
Pince dried marjoram
1/4 tsp salt
2 tbsp lemon juice
1/2 cup jack cheese, grated

Rub garlic on inside of a large salad bowl. Place vegetables in bowl and gently toss the olive oil through them. This coats the vegetables and keeps the salad from becoming limp.

Now add the seasonings, lemon juice, and cheese. Again, toss gently, being careful not to overstir.

Makes 4 servings. This salad is rich in vitamins A and C, riboflavin, and folic acid.

You may wish to add more cheese and serve it as the main dish for lunch or a light supper. Accompany with whole-grain bread or rolls.

EACH SERVING PROVIDES
159 calories
8 g protein
12 g fat
16 mg cholesterol

OR EXCHANGES AS FOLLOWS
1 vegetable
1 meat
2 fat

CARROT-RAISIN-PINEAPPLE SALAD (QUICK)

1 tsp grated orange peel
Dash nutmeg
4 cups carrots (about 6 large),
   finely grated

Combine the orange peel, nutmeg, carrots, pineapple (including juice), and raisins. Refrigerate, if possible, for a

1 (8-3/4 oz) can crushed
  pineapple (in own juice)
1/2 cup raisins, packed

few hours in order to blend the flavors.

Makes 8 servings. Stores well in the refrigerator for several days.

CALIFORNIA DREAMIN' SALAD (QUICK)

1 large carrot, coarsely grated
1 medium apple, coarsely
  grated
2 ribs celery, finely chopped
5 radishes, grated
1 cup red cabbage, shredded
1/4 cup parsley, minced
1/4 cup raisins
2 tbsp sunflower seeds
4 leaves romaine lettuce
1/8 cup safflower oil
2-3 tbsp lemon juice
1/2 tsp honey
1/8 tsp salt

Combine the carrots, apples, celery, radishes, cabbage, parsley, raisins, and sunflower seeds.

Mix the oil, lemon juice, honey, and salt. Toss through the vegetable-fruit mixture.

Serve at once on individual romaine leaves. Makes 4 servings.

MIXED VEGETABLE COLESLAW

1/4 head red cabbage, finely
  shredded
1/4 head green cabbage, finely
  shredded
1 red (or green) pepper, seeded
  and chopped
2 ribs celery, thinly sliced
4 green onions, thinly sliced
2 large carrots, grated
1/3 cup Creamy Yogurt
  Dressing

Prepare the vegetables. Combine in a large salad bowl. Add dressing and blend gently.

Salad may be served immediately or it can be refrigerated for a few hours.

Makes 4 servings.

EACH SERVING PROVIDES
117 calories
4 g protein
6 g fat
17 g carbohydrate
8 mg cholesterol

OR EXCHANGES AS FOLLOWS
3 vegetables
1 fat

CURRIED SALMON SALAD

1 (7 3/4 oz) can salmon
4 cups cooked brown rice
1/3 cup (2) green onions, sliced
2 tbsp olive oil
1 1/2 tsp curry powder
1 tbsp lemon juice
3 tbsp cider vinegar
1/4 tsp garlic powder
1 medium tomato, cut into
  wedges
Lettuce
Lemon and parsley for garnish
Condiments

Drain salmon, reserving liquid. Flake salmon and combine with rice and reserved salmon liquid.

Sauté green onion in oil with curry powder. Blend in lemon juice, vinegar, and garlic powder.

Pour dressing over salmon and rice mixture and blend thoroughly.

Pack mixture into a 1 1/2 quart round bowl lined with plastic wrap or foil. Refrigerate several hours to blend flavors.

EACH SERVING PROVIDES
352 calories
16 g protein
13 g fat

43 g carbohydrate
35 mg cholesterol

Unmold onto lettuce-lined platter. Arrange tomatoes around salad. Garnish with lemon slices and parsley.

Serve with a selection of condiments, such as chopped cucumber, seived hard-boiled egg, and chopped, toasted almonds.

Makes 4 servings. Good as leftovers for your lunch sack.

GREEK CHICKEN RICE SALAD (QUICK)

4 cups cooked brown rice,
  chilled
8 oz plain lowfat yogurt
1/4 cup mayonnaise
1/4 tsp garlic powder
1/8 tsp salt
2 cups cooked chicken, diced
1 cup celery, sliced
1/4 lb fresh spinach, cut into
  thin strips
4 green onions, sliced thinly
1 medium tomato, chopped
Lettuce
12 ripe olives for garnish

Mix the yogurt, mayonnaise, garlic powder, and salt. Add to rice and mix well. Chill until ready to serve.

Add chicken, celery, spinach, green onions, and tomato. Toss lightly.

Serve on lettuce. Garnish with olives. Makes 4 servings.

EACH SERVING PROVIDES
443 calories
25 g protein
16 g fat
52 g carbohydrate
5 mg cholesterol

OR EXCHANGES AS FOLLOWS
1 vegetable
3 bread
2 meat
2 fat

TOMATO ASPIC

3 2/3 cups tomato juice
1/2 medium onion, sliced thinly
3 stalks celery, sliced thinly
1/4 cup celery leaves
2 lemon slices
1 sprig parsley
3 peppercorns
2 cloves
1 bay leaf
1/8 tsp marjoram
1 tsp sugar
1/4 tsp salt
2 envelopes unflavored gelatin
1/4 cup vinegar
1 1/2 cups cabbage, shredded
(or any combination of fresh
vegetables)

EACH SERVING PROVIDES
13 calories
1 g protein
0 g fat
3 g carbohydrate
0 mg cholesterol

OR EXCHANGES AS FOLLOWS
Free

Combine 3 cups of the tomato juice with the onion, celery, celery leaves, lemon, parsley, peppercorns, cloves, bay leaf, marjoram, sugar, and salt. Simmer, uncovered for 10 minutes. Strain.

Meanwhile, mix the remaining juice with the vinegar. Sprinkle the gelatin over this mixture and allow it to soften. Then stir it into the hot mixture until all gelatin dissolves.

Refrigerate, stirring occasionally, until it becomes the consistency of unheated egg white. Then fold in the cabbage. Pour into a wet mold. Chill in refrigerator until thoroughly set. Unmold onto a chilled platter covered with greens. Garnish each portion with a dab of sour cream. Serves 8.

CELERY VICTOR

1 14-oz can chicken stock
1/2 medium onion, sliced
1/2 cup celery leaves
1 sprig parsley
3 peppercorns
2 cloves
1/8 tsp ground marjoram
4 celery hearts (or 8 large outer
stems, cut into 4 pieces each)
1/2 cup herb dressing
Pimento strips

Add the onion, celery leaves, parsley, peppercorns, cloves, and marjoram to the chicken stock. Bring stock to a boil. Add celery and simmer, covered, until celery is barely tender. Drain the celery, reserving the stock for gravy some other time. Marinate the celery in the salad dressing for 8 to 12 hours or overnight. Turn it a few times to

EACH SERVING PROVIDES
46 calories
0 g protein
4 g fat
3 g carbohydrate
0 mg cholesterol

OR EXCHANGES AS FOLLOWS
1/2 vegetable
1 fat

make sure that the celery remains covered with dressing.

Before serving, drain the dressing from the celery (save it for another salad). Serve the celery on a bed of lettuce. Garnish with a pimento strip. Serves 4.

LOW-CALORIE MOCK FRENCH DRESSING

1/2 cup catsup
3/4 cup rice* or cider vinegar
1/4 tsp garlic powder
1/8 tsp basil
1/8 tsp marjoram
1 tbsp oil
1 tsp sugar

EACH TABLESPOON PROVIDES
14 calories
0 g protein
1 g fat
2 g carbohydrate
0 mg cholesterol

OR EXCHANGES AS FOLLOWS
Free

Mix all ingredients together. Best to roll the herbs in your hand before adding them in order to release their flavor. (This is unnecessary if the herbs are already ground.)

Store in refrigerator.

*Rice vinegar is preferred because it is so mild in flavor.

CREAMY YOGURT DRESSING

1/8 cup unflavored lowfat yogurt
1/8 cup mayonnaise
1/8 tsp dry mustard
1/8 tsp garlic powder
1/8 tsp dill weed
1/8 tsp salt
Juice of 1 lemon

Blend all ingredients. A very small wire whisk works best to blend. Best to use within one day, as it tends to separate if left in the refrigerator longer.

EACH TABLESPOON PROVIDES
38 calories
1 g protein
4 g fat
1 g carbohydrate
6 mg cholesterol

OR EXCHANGES AS FOLLOWS
1 fat

HERB DRESSING

1 cup apple cider vinegar
1/2 tsp dry mustard
1/4 tsp black pepper
Dash cayenne (optional)
1/4 tsp basil
1/2 tsp marjoram
1/8 tsp thyme
1/8 tsp rosemary
1 tsp sugar
3/4 tsp salt
1/4 tsp garlic powder
1/4 tsp onion powder
1 cup olive oil

Mix all seasonings into the vinegar, then blend in the oil. Do not refrigerate, as olive oil will solidify.

EACH TABLESPOON PROVIDES
63 calories
0 g protein
7 g fat
0 g carbohydrate
0 mg cholesterol

OR EXCHANGES AS FOLLOWS
1 1/2 fat

LEMON SALAD DRESSING

1/4 cup fresh lemon juice
1/2 tsp salt
1/8 tsp pepper
1/2 tsp sugar
1/4 tsp dry mustard
1/2 cup corn or safflower oil

EACH TABLESPOON PROVIDES
84 calories
0 g protein
9 g fat
1 g carbohydrate
0 mg cholesterol

OR EXCHANGES AS FOLLOWS
2 fat

Beat together the first 5 ingredients. Then beat in the oil in a slow and steady stream.

For Your
Sweet Tooth

ALMOND-PEAR TORTE WITH ORANGE SAUCE

2 cups chopped pears (about 2
    large pears)
1/2 cup butter or margarine, at
    room temperature
1/2 cup granulated sugar
1/4 cup brown sugar, firmly
    packed
2 eggs
1 tsp vanilla
1/2 tsp almond extract
1 cup all-purpose flour
1 cup whole wheat pastry flour
2 tsp soda
1 tsp ground cinnamon
1/2 tsp ground nutmeg
1/4 tsp ground cloves
1/2 cup raisins
Orange Sauce

ORANGE SAUCE
2 tbsp cornstarch
1/2 cup sugar
2 tsp orange rind, grated finely
1/2 tsp almond extract
2 cups water
1/4 cup orange juice

EACH SERVING PROVIDES
276 calories
4 g protein
9 g fat
47 g carbohydrate
66 mg cholesterol

OR EXCHANGES AS FOLLOWS
2 bread
2 fat
5 tsp sugar

Core and finely chop pears. In a large bowl, beat together the butter and sugar until creamy. Add the eggs, one at a time, beating well after each addition until light and fluffy. Blend in vanilla, almond extract, and pears. In a separate bowl, stir together flours, soda, and spices. Add this flour mixture to pear mixture and blend thoroughly. Stir in raisins. Pour into a well-greased spring-bottom tube pan or a 2-quart tube mold. Bake at 350°F for 60 minutes, or until a wooden pick inserted in center comes out clean. Cool in pan for 20 minutes and then turn out onto a wire rack. Cool thoroughly. Serve with Orange Sauce. Serves 12.

To make sauce, mix cornstarch, sugar, orange rind, almond extract and water together in a saucepan. Stir over low heat until sauce thickens. Remove from heat and add orange juice. Serve 1/8 cup sauce with each slice of torte.

APPLE CAKE

3 cups tart apples, diced
1/2 cup walnuts, chopped
1 cup whole-wheat pastry flour
1 tsp baking soda
1/2 tsp cinnamon
1/4 tsp nutmeg
1/2 cup sugar
3 tbsp butter
1 egg
1 tsp vanilla

EACH SERVING PROVIDES
224 calories
4 g protein
5 g fat
38 g carbohydrate
44 mg cholesterol

OR EXCHANGES AS FOLLOWS
1 1/2 bread
1 fat
3 tsp sugar

Cut apples into small chunks, leaving the skins on. Chop walnuts. Mix the flour, soda and spices. Cream sugar and butter. Add egg and vanilla. Then blend in the flour mixture. Add the apples and walnuts. (Dough will be stiff.) Spread mixture in an ungreased 9" × 9" pan and bake at 350°F for 45 minutes. Serves 8.

This recipe can be used as a dessert or as a breakfast bread. It's more nourishing than most coffee cakes. Great for morning meeting refreshments.

CARROT-PINEAPPLE CAKE

1 1/2 cups whole-wheat pastry
  flour
1/2 cup sugar
1/2 tsp baking powder
1 tsp baking soda
1 tsp cinnamon
1/4 tsp salt
1/2 cup oil
2 eggs
1 cup finely grated carrot, not
  packed (about 4 oz)
1 8-oz can crushed pineapple,
  drained to make 2/3 cup
1 tsp vanilla

Stir together the flour, sugar, baking powder, soda, cinnamon, and salt. Add the oil, eggs, carrot, pineapple and vanilla and mix until moistened. Beat 2 minutes with electric mixer.

Bake in a greased 9" × 9" × 2" pan at 350°F for 35 to 40 minutes or until cake springs back when touched lightly with finger.

Cool 10 minutes. Remove from pan and sprinkle with powdered sugar. Serves 9.

Very light and moist, and contains about half as much fat as most carrot cake recipes.

ITALIAN CHEESE CAKE

1 tbsp butter or margarine
4 graham crackers, crumbled
1 1/2 cups ricotta cheese
2 eggs
1/4 cup sugar
1/8 tsp salt
2 tbsp brandy
1 tsp almond extract
1/2 cup raisins, chopped
1 tsp cinnamon
1 tbsp sugar

EACH SERVING PROVIDES
191 calories
7 g protein
9 g fat
21 g carbohydrate
82 mg cholesterol

OR EXCHANGES AS FOLLOWS
1 1/2 fruit
1 meat
1 fat
2 tsp sugar

Rub bottom and sides of a 9" pie plate with butter. If there's any butter left, melt it and mix with crumbs. Now sprinkle crumbs into plate, turning it to coat bottom and sides.

Rub ricotta against sides of mixing bowl to remove lumps. Add eggs, sugar, salt, brandy, almond extract, and raisins. Mix thoroughly. Pour carefully into pie plate. Bake in 450°F oven 15 minutes. Then reduce heat to 325°F for another 20 minutes. Remove from oven and sprinkle with cinnamon and sugar. Serve at room temperature or cold. Serves 8.

VARIATION: Instead of brandy and almond extract, you can add the grated rinds of 1 orange and 1 lemon, plus 1 tsp each orange and lemon juice.

NOTE: A comparable serving of standard cheese cake made with cream cheese and sour cream contains 530 calories, 9 g protein, 37 g fat, 42 g carbohydrate, 131 mg cholesterol.

CINNAMON TREAT (QUICK)

1 slice whole-wheat bread
1 tsp butter or margarine
1 tsp brown sugar
Cinnamon to taste
1 tbsp raisins

EACH SERVING PROVIDES
137 calories
2 g protein
5 g fat
23 g carbohydrate
12 mg cholesterol

OR EXCHANGES AS FOLLOWS
1/2 fruit
1 bread
1 fat
1 tsp sugar

Toast bread and butter lightly. Sprinkle sugar and then cinnamon onto bread and top with raisins.

Delicious and satisfying for a late evening snack. Also a more nutritious alternative to donuts or coffee-cake in the morning.

NOTE: An iced donut provides 151 calories, 2 g protein, 7 g fat, 22 g carbohydrate. An iced coffeecake provides 346 calories, 3 g protein, 9 g fat, 67 g carbohydrate.

BRANDIED PUMPKIN CUSTARD

3 cups whole milk
5/8 cup sugar
3/8 cup brandy
1 16-oz can pumpkin
6 eggs, lightly beaten
Nutmeg

EACH SERVING (IF MADE WITH WHOLE MILK) PROVIDES
108 calories
6 g protein
5 g fat
15 g carbohydrate
123 mg cholesterol

OR EXCHANGES AS FOLLOWS
1/2 milk
1 fat
2 tsp sugar

Preheat oven to 325°F. Scald milk and beat in sugar, brandy, and pumpkin. Beat some of this hot mixture into eggs. Return all to saucepan. Beat until blended in warm saucepan, but do not return to heat. Fill custard cups. Set in shallow baking dish and place in oven. Fill pan with hot water to within 3/4" from top of cups. Bake at 325°F for 45 to 60 minutes, or until knife inserted in center comes out clean. (This usually takes a full 60 minutes.) Makes 13 half-cup servings.

You may wish to substitute half-and-half for the whole milk to make a richer custard. Better not to do this, however, unless you have planned a very lowfat meal to accompany this richer custard. Each serving of half-and-half version provides 164 calories, 5 g protein, 9 g fat, 15 g carbohydrate, 136 mg cholesterol. Exchanges remain the same, except that you must add another fat.

GAELIC GINGER CAKE

1/3 cup oil
1/3 cup dark brown sugar, packed
2 eggs
1 cup boiling water
1/2 cup blackstrap molasses
1/2 cup rolled oats, uncooked
1 1/2 cups whole-wheat pastry flour
1/2 tsp cinnamon
1 tsp ginger
1/8 tsp nutmeg
1/8 tsp cloves
1/2 tsp soda
1 1/2 tsp baking powder
1/8 tsp salt
1 tbsp grated lemon peel

EACH SERVING PROVIDES
238 calories
5 g protein
10 g fat
35 g carbohydrate
56 mg cholesterol

OR EXCHANGES AS FOLLOWS
2 bread
2 fat
1/2 tsp sugar

Heat oven to 350°F. Grease a 9" square pan. Combine oil, sugar, and eggs. Beat well. Blend in boiling water, molasses, and oats. Add all the rest of the ingredients. Mix well. Bake for 45 minutes. Top with powdered sugar. Serves 9.

This cake looks like a rich devil's food cake, but it's far healthier. Each piece provides iron equivalent to amount found in 2 to 3 oz cooked red meat and calcium equivalent to amount found in 1/3 cup milk.

BAKED RICE CUSTARD

2 cups whole milk
2 eggs, beaten
1/4 tsp salt
1/3 cup sugar
1 1/2 cups cooked brown rice
1/2 cup raisins, plumped in hot
    water and then drained
1 tsp vanilla
1/8 tsp cinnamon
Nutmeg

EACH SERVING PROVIDES
157 calories
5 g protein
4 g fat
26 g carbohydrate
71 mg cholesterol

OR EXCHANGES AS FOLLOWS
1/2 milk
1 bread
1 fat
1 tsp sugar

Scald milk. Combine eggs, salt, and sugar in a bowl. Gradually add hot milk, then stir in rice, raisins, vanilla, and cinnamon. Turn into individual baking dishes and sprinkle tops with a little nutmeg.

Place dishes in a shallow pan containing about an inch of water. Bake at 325°F for 1 hour or until almost firm.

Makes 8 (1/2 cup) servings.

BAKED PEARS WITH LEMON SAUCE

PEARS
4 large firm pears
1 tbsp honey
2 1/2 tbsp water
2 whole cloves

LEMON SAUCE
1 tbsp cornstarch
1 1/2 cups nonfat milk
1/2 tsp ground cinnamon
2 tsp grated lemon rind
1/4 cup lemon juice
2 tbsp honey

EACH SERVING PROVIDES
110 calories
3 g protein

Cut pears in half and remove cores. Arrange pears in a glass baking dish. Heat the honey, water, and cloves in a small pan, but do not boil. Pour over the pears. Bake until tender, about 20 to 30 minutes.

Meanwhile, dissolve cornstarch in a little of the milk in a saucepan. Add remaining milk and cinnamon. Cook over medium-low heat, stirring, until mixture thickens. Add lemon rind, lemon juice, and honey. This can be made ahead of time and stored covered

Trace fat
26 g carbohydrate
0 mg cholesterol

OR EXCHANGES AS FOLLOWS
1/2 milk
2 fruit

in the refrigerator. It may be served
hot or cold.

Serve 1/4 cup sauce over each warm
pear half. Makes 8 servings.

STEAMED PERSIMMON PUDDING WITH LEMON SAUCE

3 large ripe persimmons
1 cup whole wheat pastry flour
1/4 tsp salt
1 1/2 tsp soda
1/2 tsp cinnamon
1/2 cup sugar
1 egg, well-beaten
2 tbsp melted butter or oil
3/4 cup lowfat milk
1 tsp vanilla
1/2 cup raisins
Lemon sauce

LEMON SAUCE
1 tbsp cornstarch
1/4 cup sugar
Grated peel from 1 lemon
1 cup water
2 tbsp lemon juice
1 tbsp butter or margarine

EACH SERVING PROVIDES
249 calories
5 g protein
6 g fat
48 g carbohydrate
47 mg cholesterol

OR EXCHANGES AS FOLLOWS
1/2 fruit
2 bread
1 fat
4 tsp sugar

To prepare the pudding, cut the persimmons in halves. Peel and remove
the fibrous section in the center. Mash
the pulp. Measure out the flour and
add to it the salt, soda, and cinnamon.
Set aside.

Now add the sugar, egg, butter, milk,
vanilla, and flour mixture to the persimmons. Beat to a thin batter. Stir in
the raisins. Turn into a greased 8" casserole, cover tightly and bake at 350°F
for 1 hour.

Best served warm with hot lemon
sauce, but also good cold. Serves 8.

To prepare the lemon sauce, combine
the cornstarch, sugar, lemon peel, and
water in a saucepan. Stir over low
heat until the sauce is thickened. Remove from heat. Blend in the lemon
juice and butter.

Sensational! Moist. Tastes rich but is
very low in fat. Men love it.

RASPBERRY BAVARIAN

1 envelope plain gelatin
1/4 cup cold water
1 10-oz pkg frozen raspberries
1 cup lowfat yogurt, unflavored
2 egg whites

EACH SERVING PROVIDES
122 calories
6 g protein
2 g fat
21 g carbohydrate
3 mg cholesterol

OR EXCHANGES AS FOLLOWS
1 meat
2 fruit

Soak gelatin in cold water. Drain fruit well. Reserve 3/4 cup of juice, adding water if necessary to make 3/4 cup. Stir gelatin mixture into juice over medium heat until gelatin is dissolved. Then add fruit and chill. Whip egg white until peaks form. When gelatin mixture begins to thicken, fold in yogurt and then egg white. Pile into parfait (or wine) glasses. Garnish with a few slivered almonds. Serves 4.

Most frozen raspberries already have sugar added. If you do not use sweetened berries, this recipe will be much too sour.

SUNSET MELON BOWL

2 cantaloupes, cut into balls
Juice of 1/2 lemon
1 carton fresh* blueberries, cleaned
1 10-oz pkg frozen raspberries, sweetened and thawed
1/4 cup Creme de Cassis liqueur

EACH SERVING PROVIDES
109 calories
1 g protein
0 g fat
24 g carbohydrate
0 mg cholesterol

OR EXCHANGES AS FOLLOWS
2 1/2 fruit

Cut cantaloupe into balls and mix with lemon juice. Add blueberries.

Purée the raspberries in blender. Then strain out all the seeds, preferably through cheesecloth placed in a strainer. (We tried leaving the seeds for extra fiber, but the flavor was adversely affected).

Now mix raspberry purée and liqueur into cantaloupe and blueberry mixture. Allow to sit in refrigerator for several hours before serving in order for the flavors to blend. Serves 8. Colors of a sumptuous sunset.

*May substitute 2 cups blueberries, frozen with no added sugar.

FRUIT WITH YOGURT SAUCE

2 cups unflavored lowfat yogurt
1 1/2 tbsp mild honey
1 tsp vanilla extract
1/2 tsp almond extract
3 cups fruit pieces

EACH SERVING PROVIDES
142 calories
6 g protein
3 g fat
26 g carbohydrate
6 mg cholesterol

OR EXCHANGES AS FOLLOWS
1/2 milk
1 1/2 fruit
1 tsp sugar

Mix the yogurt, honey, and flavorings until smooth. Pour over sliced fresh or frozen (without sugar) fruit. Peaches, bananas, cherries, or berries are especially good with this sauce. Serves 4.

A tasty and more nourishing substitute for an ice cream sundae.

BANANAS IN SOUR CREAM SAUCE

1/2 cup unflavored lowfat yogurt
1/2 cup sour cream
2 tbsp real maple syrup
1 tsp vanilla
2 medium bananas

EACH SERVING PROVIDES
163 calories
3 g protein
7 g fat
25 g carbohydrate
18 mg cholesterol

OR EXCHANGES AS FOLLOWS
1/2 milk
1 1/2 fruit
1 1/4 fat
1 tsp sugar

Blend yogurt, sour cream, maple syrup, and vanilla. Slice bananas into wine glasses, drizzling sauce throughout. Garnish with a berry or fresh mint. Serves 4.

Also good with fresh peaches or any type of fresh or frozen berry.

AMBROSIA

1 8-oz can crushed pineapple
(canned in own juice)
1/2 cup walnuts
1 lb seedless grapes
2 oranges
1 16-oz carton unflavored lowfat
yogurt

EACH SERVING PROVIDES
134 calories
4 g protein
5 g fat
20 g carbohydrate
4 mg cholesterol

OR EXCHANGES AS FOLLOWS
1/2 milk
1 1/2 fruit
1 fat

Drain pineapple (reserve juice for beverage or gelatin dessert). Chop walnuts. Clean grapes. Peel and section oranges and then cut each section in half. Mix fruit and nuts into yogurt. Store in refrigerator for a few hours before serving, so flavors have a chance to combine. Serves 8.

BANANA-PINEAPPLE-ORANGE SMOOTHIE (QUICK)

1 large banana, frozen
1 (7 3/4-oz) can crushed
pineapple, canned in its own
juice, chilled
1 cup orange juice, chilled
Mint sprigs for garnish

EACH SERVING PROVIDES
92 calories
2 g protein
0 g fat
23 g carbohydrate
0 mg cholesterol

OR EXCHANGES AS FOLLQWS
2 fruit

Peel banana and slice into a few large pieces. Place banana, pineapple (along with its juice), and orange juice in blender jar. Blend until smooth.

Makes 4 servings. Garnish with fresh mint sprigs.

Very refreshing. Has the consistency of a thick milkshake, but lower in calories and contains no fat.

BERRY SMOOTH (QUICK)

1 large banana, frozen
1 cup fresh or frozen berries or
cherries

Peel banana and slice into a few large pieces. Purée banana and berries or cherries in blender until smooth.

EACH SERVING PROVIDES
120 calories
1 g protein
0 g fat
20 g carbohydrate
0 mg cholesterol

Makes 2 servings.

If you use frozen berries, be sure to purchase those without added sugar.

OR EXCHANGES AS FOLLOWS
3 fruit

TROPICAL FRUIT SAUCE (QUICK)

1/2 large banana
1 large mango
2 tbsp orange juice
1/2 tsp lime rind

Peel banana. Peel and seed mango, then chop it coarsely. Grate lime. Blenderize all ingredients until smooth.

EACH SERVING PROVIDES
66 calories
Trace protein
Trace fat
18 g carbohydrate
0 mg cholesterol

Serve over fresh fruit or a small scoop of vanilla ice cream.

Makes 4 servings.

OR EXCHANGES AS FOLLOWS
1 1/2 fruit

Dips, Spreads, and Sauces

GARBANZO DIP (MOCK GUACAMOLE)

1/4 cup onion, chopped
1 tbsp olive oil
1/3 cup parsley, chopped
1/4 tsp salt
1/2 tsp basil
1/8 tsp ground oregano
1/8 tsp ground cumin
1 small clove garlic, crushed
1/4 cup lemon juice
1/4 cup bean juice
1 15-oz can garbanzo beans, drained
3 tbsp tahini*

EACH SERVING PROVIDES
87 calories
3 g protein
5 g fat
9 g carbohydrate
0 mg cholesterol

OR EXCHANGES AS FOLLOWS
2 vegetable
1 fat

Mix onion, oil, parsley, salt, basil, oregano, cumin, garlic, and lemon juice with the bean juice in a blender until puréed. Add the garbanzo beans slowly, blending until smooth after each addition. Blend in the tahini.

Serve with assorted fresh vegetables as a dip. It's sensational. Also makes a nourishing and tasty lunch served with whole-grain bread for dipping. Makes approximately 2 cups or 8 (1/4 cup) servings.

This dip looks like guacamole, but is much lower in fat and really delicious.

*Tahini is sesame seed paste, a Middle Eastern staple. It is available in vacuum-packed cans or jars at most natural food stores and some markets.

TUNA DIP-SPREAD

1 7 1/2-oz can tuna, drained of oil
3/4 cup lowfat cottage cheese or buttermilk
1/8 tsp garlic powder
2 tsp lemon juice

Combine tuna, cottage cheese, garlic powder, lemon juice, celery seed, and parsley in blender container. Blend until smooth. Makes approximately 2 cups or 8 (1/4) cup servings.

1/4 tsp celery seed
1/4 cup chopped parsley

Serve with assorted fresh vegetables and/or whole-grain crackers or bread.

EGGPLANT DIP–SPREAD I

1 large eggplant, diced
6 tbsp olive oil
1 clove garlic, crushed
1 cup celery, diced
1 green pepper, seeded & diced
1 8-oz can tomato purée
1/8 tsp cayenne pepper
1 tbsp ground cumin
2 tbsp brown sugar
1 tsp salt
1/4 cup apple cider vinegar
2/3 cup chopped parsley

Cut eggplant into 1/2″ cubes. Prepare the rest of the vegetables. Now heat 4 tbsp oil in a large skillet and sauté the eggplant cubes until golden brown over medium heat, stirring often to prevent sticking. Remove to a bowl and cover to continue steaming while you cook the garlic, celery, and green pepper in the remaining 2 tbsp oil.

Meanwhile, mix the tomato purée, cayenne, cumin, sugar, salt, and vinegar. When the green pepper and celery are barely tender, add the eggplant and tomato mixture to the skillet. Cover and simmer for 30 minutes or longer, stirring occasionally to prevent sticking.

Cover and chill dip overnight. Just before serving, mix in the parsley. Serve with whole-grain crackers or pita bread cut into small wedges. Makes approximately 4 cups or 16 (1/4 cup) servings.

Also good as a main dish. Thin with a little water or tomato juice and serve over spaghetti. Garnish with grated mozzarella cheese.

EGGPLANT DIP–SPREAD II

1 large eggplant, diced
2 medium onions, diced
1 large green pepper, diced
3 cloves garlic, crushed
1/4 cup olive oil
1 15-oz can tomatoes
1/2 tsp salt
1/8 tsp pepper
1 tbsp Worcestershire sauce
1 cup lowfat yogurt
2 tbsp lemon juice
2/3 cup parsley, minced
1/2 6-oz can tomato paste

EACH SERVING PROVIDES
66 calories
2 g protein
4 g fat
6 g carbohydrate
1 mg cholesterol

OR EXCHANGES AS FOLLOWS
1 vegetable
1 fat

Prepare the vegetables. Heat oil in a large skillet. Sauté eggplant, onions, green pepper, and garlic over medium heat until the onions are translucent. Stir occasionally to prevent the vegetables from sticking.

Lower the heat and add the tomatoes. Cook until the vegetables are tender, again stirring occasionally.

Cool to lukewarm. Stir in the salt, pepper, Worchestershire sauce, yogurt, lemon juice, parsley, and tomato paste. Chill in the refrigerator until ready to serve.

Garnish with additional chopped parsley and serve with whole-grain crackers. Makes approximately 1 quart or 16 (1/4 cup) servings.

LOW-CALORIE MUSHROOM SAUCE

2 cups mushrooms, chopped
1 tbsp soy sauce
1/2 cup onion, chopped
1 14-oz can beef or chicken broth

EACH SERVING PROVIDES
43 calories
4 g protein

Combine the mushrooms, soy sauce, onion, and broth in a small saucepan. Cook over medium heat until mushrooms are tender. Purée in blender until smooth.

Serve over cooked meat, fish, or poultry. Also nice over rice.

0 g fat
6 g carbohydrate
0 mg cholesterol

Makes approximately 1 cup or 4 (1/4 cup) servings.

ITALIAN TOMATO SAUCE

1/4 cup olive oil
2 cups onions, diced
4 large cloves garlic, minced
2 large green peppers, diced
4 bay leaves
2 vegetable bouillon cubes
2 29-oz cans tomato puree
1/2 tsp rosemary
1/2 tsp thyme
1 tsp oregano
1 tsp basil

EACH SERVING PROVIDES
156 calories
4 g protein
7 g fat
22 g carbohydrate
0 mg cholesterol

OR EXCHANGES AS FOLLOWS
1 vegetable
1 bread
1/2 fat

Sauté onions and garlic in oil until the onions are translucent. Add all the rest of the ingredients. If the herbs are not already ground, crush them in your hands to help release the flavor. Simmer the mixture for 30 minutes or longer.

Makes approximately 8 (1 cup) servings.

Prepare a double batch. This sauce freezes well.

LOW-CALORIE GRAVY JARDINIÈRE

1/4 cup onion, chopped
1/2 cup celery, chopped
1/3 cup carrot, chopped
3 tbsp parsley, chopped
1/8 tsp herb salt or poultry
seasoning
1/4 tsp ground thyme
Pinch basil

Combine the onion, celery, carrot, parsley, herb salt, thyme, basil, sugar, and 1/2 cup chicken broth. Bring to a boil, then simmer until vegetables are tender.

Purée mixture in the blender, adding remaining broth as needed, until

1 tsp sugar
1 1/4 cups chicken broth
Dash pepper

smooth. Add a little pepper to taste. Reheat and serve hot over turkey slices or other meats.

Makes approximately 1 1/3 cups or 4 (1/3 cup) servings.

Appendix A: Exchange System

The exchange lists that follow are adapted from the *Exchange Lists for Meal Planning*, prepared by committees of the American Diabetes Association, Inc., and The American Dietetic Association in cooperation with

The National Institute of Arthritis, Metabolism, and Digestive Diseases
National Heart and Lung Institute
National Institutes of Health, Public Health Service
U.S. Department of Health, Education, and Welfare.

We have added the number of servings from each list which were recommended for the Sample Weight-Loss Plans explained in Chapter 14, "When You're Weigh Off Balance."

TABLE A-1. **Milk exchanges.**

Emphasize nonfat or lowfat varieties.	One exchange (serving size as listed) of nonfat milk supplies approximately: 80 calories 8 g protein 0 g fat* 12 g carbohydrate

1200 Calorie Plan—include 1 Milk Exchange daily**
1500 Calorie Plan—include 1 1/2 Milk Exchanges daily**
1800 Calorie Plan—include 2 Milk Exchanges daily**

NONFAT MILK GROUP:

Skim or nonfat milk	1 cup	
Powdered nonfat dry milk (solids only)	1/3 cup	
Canned, evaporated nonfat milk	1/2 cup	
Buttermilk made from nonfat milk	1 cup	
Yogurt (unflavored) made from nonfat milk	1 cup	

LOWFAT MILK:

1% fat milk	1 cup	(+ 1/2 fat exchange)
2% fat milk	1 cup	(+ 1 fat exchange)
Yogurt (unflavored) made from 2% milk	1 cup	(+ 1 fat exchange)

WHOLE MILK GROUP:

Whole milk	1 cup	(+ 2 fat exchanges)
Canned, evaporated whole milk	1/2 cup	(+ 2 fat exchanges)
Buttermilk made from whole milk	1 cup	(+ 2 fat exchanges)
Yogurt (unflavored) made from whole milk	1 cup	(+ 2 fat exchanges)

* When you use fat-containing milk or milk products, count the fat(s) as part of the Fat Exchange servings alloted to your calorie level.
** The amount of milk specified for the calorie levels above may not supply you with enough calcium, particularly if you are a teenager. It would be a good idea to eat extra calcium-rich foods (see Chapter 17) and/or to include one to two ounces of cheese as part of your Meat Exchanges.

TABLE A-2. **Vegetable exchanges.**

Emphasize dark green leafy and deep orange varieties.	One exchange (serving of 1/2 cup) supplies approximately 25 calories 2 g protein 0 g fat 5 g carbohydrate

1200 Calorie Plan—include 3 Vegetable Exchanges daily*
1500 Calorie Plan—include 4 Vegetable Exchanges daily*
1800 Calorie Plan—include 5 Vegetable Exchanges daily*

Artichokes
Asparagus
Bean sprouts
Beets
Bok choy
Broccoli
Brussel sprouts
Cabbage
Carrots
Cauliflower
Chard
Chicory
Cilantro
Celery
Cucumbers
Endive
Escarole
Eggplant
Green pepper
Greens:
  Beet
  Collard
  Dandelion
  Kale

Greens:
  Mustard
  Turnip
Jicama
Lettuce
Mint
Mushrooms
Okra
Onions
Parsley
Radishes
Rhubarb
Rutabaga
Sauerkraut
Spinach
String beans, green or yellow
Summer squash
Tomatoes
Tomato juice
Turnips
Vegetable juice cocktail
Watercress
Zucchini

*These vegetables may actually be eaten as desired because they are so low in calories. They're also good sources of fiber. Starchy vegetables are listed on the Bread Exchange list.

150

TABLE A-3. **Fruit exchanges.**

Emphasize those rich in vitamin C and try to use whole fruits rather than juice for fiber.	One exchange (serving size as listed) provides approximately 40 calories 0 g protein 0 g fat 10 g carbohydrate

1200 Calorie Plan—include 3 Fruit Exchanges daily
1500 Calorie Plan—include 4 Fruit Exchanges daily
1800 Calorie Plan—include 4 Fruit Exchanges daily

All fruits and juices are most nutritious if eaten fresh or prepared without the addition of sugar.

Apple	1 small	Mango	1/2 small
Apple juice	1/3 cup	Melon:	
Applesauce	1/2 cup	Cantaloupe	1/4 medium
Apricots, fresh	2 medium	Honeydew	1/8 medium
Apricots, dried	4 halves	Watermelon	1 cup
Banana	1/2 small	Nectarine	1 small
Berries:		Orange	1 small
Blackberries	1/2 cup	Orange juice	1/2 cup
Blueberries	1/2 cup	Papaya	3/4 cup
Raspberries	1/2 cup	Peach	1 medium
Strawberries	3/4 cup	Pear	1 small
Cherries	10 large	Persimmon	1 medium
Cider	1/3 cup	Pineapple	1/2 cup
Cranberry juice	1/4 cup	Pineapple juice	1/3 cup
Dates	2	Plums	2 medium
Figs, fresh	1	Prunes	2 medium
Figs, dried	1	Prune juice	1/4 cup
Grapefruit	1/2	Raisins	2 tbsp
Grapefruit juice	1/2 cup	Tangerine	1 medium
Grapes	12	Other, unsweetened	1/2 cup
Grape juice	1/4 cup		

TABLE A-4. **Bread exchanges.**

Emphasize whole-grain breads and cereals.	One exchange (serving size as listed) supplies approximately 70 calories 2 g protein 0 g fat 15 g carbohydrate

1200 Calorie Plan—include 6 Bread Exchanges daily
1500 Calorie Plan—include 7 Bread Exchanges daily
1800 Calorie Plan—include 9 Bread Exchanges daily

BREADS:

Bagel	1/2
Bread	1 slice
Bread crumbs, dried	3 tbsp
English muffin	1/2
Roll, dinner	1
Roll, hamburger or hot dog	1/2
Tortilla, 6″	1

CEREALS:

Bran flakes	1/2 cup
Cereals, other ready-to-eat unsweetened	1/2 cup
Cereal, puffed (unfrosted)	1 cup
Cereal, cooked	1/2 cup
Cornmeal, dry	2 tbsp
Flour	2 1/2 tbsp
Pasta, cooked (spaghetti, noodles, macaroni)	1/2 cup
Popcorn, popped (no fat added on top)	1 cup
Popcorn, air popped	3 cups
Rice or barley, cooked	1/2 cup
Wheat germ	2 tbsp

CRACKERS:

Arrowroot	3
Graham, 2 1/2″ square	2
Matzoh, 4 × 6″	1/2
Oyster	20
Pretzels, very thin sticks, 3 1/8″	25
Rye wafers, 2 × 3 1/2″	3
Saltines	6
Soda	4

STARCHY VEGETABLES:

Corn	1/3 cup
Corn on cob	1 small
Lima beans	1/2 cup
Parsnips	2/3 cup
Peas	1/2 cup
Potato, white	1 small
Potato, mashed	1/2 cup
Pumpkin	3/4 cup
Squash, winter (Acorn, Butternut)	1/2 cup
Yam or sweet potato	1/4 cup

PRODUCTS WITH ADDED FAT:

Biscuit, 2″ diameter	1 (+ 1 fat exchange)
Corn bread, 2 × 2 × 1″	1 (+ 1 fat exchange)
Crackers, butter-type	5 (+ 1 fat exchange)
Muffin, plain	1 (+ 1 fat exchange)
Pancake, 5 × 1/2″	1 (+ 1 fat exchange)
Potatoes, french-fried	8 (+ 1 fat exchange)
Potato or corn chips	8 (+ 1 fat exchange)
Waffle, 5 × 1/2″	1 (+ 1 fat exchange)

TABLE A-5. **Meat exchanges.**

Emphasize those lowest in fat content and trim away all visible fat. Have fish, chicken and legumes more often.	One exchange (serving size as listed) supplies approximately (if from Group I) 55 calories 7 g protein 3 g fat* 0 g carbohydrate

1200 Calorie Plan—include 4 Meat Exchanges daily
1500 Calorie Plan—include 5 Meat Exchanges daily
1800 Calorie Plan—include 6 Meat Exchanges daily

GROUP I (LOWEST FAT CONTENT):

Beef:	Baby beef, chipped beef, chuck, flank steak, tenderloin, plate ribs, plate skirt steak, round (bottom and top), all cuts rump, tripe.	1 oz cooked
Cheese:	Cottage cheese, dry and lowfat	1/4 cup
Fish:	Any fresh or frozen	1 oz cooked
	Canned salmon, tuna, mackerel, crab, lobster	1/4 cup
	Clams, oysters, scallops, shrimp	5 or 1 oz
	Sardines, drained	3
Lamb:	Leg, rib, sirloin, loin (roast and chops), shank, shoulder	1 oz cooked

GROUP I (LOWEST FAT CONTENT):

Legumes:	Beans (black, kidney, pinto, soy); lentils; peas (blackeyed, split)	1/2 cup cooked (+ 1 Bread Exchange)
	Peanut butter	2 tbsp (+ 2 Fat Exchanges)
	Soybean curd (tofu)	1/3 cup
Organs:	Heart, kidney, liver	1 oz cooked
Pork:	Leg (whole rump, center shank), ham (center slices)	1 oz cooked
Poultry:	Chicken, turkey, cornish hen (no skin)	1 oz cooked
Veal:	Leg, loin, rib, shank, shoulder, cutlets (not breaded and fried)	1 oz cooked

GROUP II (MEDIUM FAT CONTENT):

Beef:	Ground (15% fat), corned beef (canned), rib eye, round (ground commercial)	1 oz cooked
Cheese:	Cottage, creamed	1/4 cup
	Mozzarella, Ricotta, Farmer's, Neufchatel	1 oz
	Parmesan	1/4 cup
Egg:		1
Organs:	Sweetbreads	1 oz cooked
Pork:	Loin (all cuts tenderloin), shoulder arm (picnic), shoulder blade, Boston butt, Canadian bacon, boiled ham	1 oz cooked

GROUP III (HIGH FAT CONTENT):

Beef:	Brisket, corned beef, ground beef (more than 20% fat), hamburger (commercial), chuck (ground commercial), roasts (rib), steaks (club and rib)	1 oz cooked
Cheese:	Cheddar, jack, others not listed in the other groups	1 oz

GROUP III (HIGH FAT CONTENT):

Deli:	Cold cuts (salami, bologna, etc.)	1 oz
	Frankfurter	1 medium
Lamb:	Breast	1 oz cooked
Pork:	Spare ribs, loin (back ribs), pork (ground), sausage, country-style ham, deviled ham	1 oz cooked
Poultry:	Capon, duck (domestic), goose	1 oz cooked
Veal:	Breast	1 oz cooked

*Groups II and III are higher in fat content and therefore supply more calories. One exchange from Group II contains approximately 75 calories. One exchange from Group III contains approximately 100 calories. You'll need to count each serving from Group II as 1 Meat Exchange and 1/2 Fat Exchange and each serving from Group III as 1 Meat Exchange and 1 Fat Exchange. Figure the added Fat Exchanges as part of those alloted to your calorie level.

TABLE A-6. **Fat exchanges.**

Emphasize a variety from natural sources. Try to avoid those containing hydrogenated fats.	One exchange (serving size as listed) supplies approximately 45 calories 0 g protein 5 g fat 0 g carbohydrate

1200 Calorie Plan—include 6 Fat Exchanges daily
1500 Calorie Plan—include 8 Fat Exchanges daily
1800 Calorie Plan—include 9 Fat Exchanges daily

POLYUNSATURATED:

Margarines: Parkay (soft safflower), Promise, Saffola	1 tsp
Mayonnaise	1 tsp
Oils: corn, cottonseed, safflower, soy, sunflower	1 tsp
Salad dressings made with polyunsaturated oils (French, Italian, mayonnaise-type)	1 tbsp
Seeds: sesame, sunflower	1 tbsp
Walnuts	6 halves

MONOUNSATURATED:

Avocado, 4″ diameter	1/8
Margarines, all except those mentioned above or below	1 tsp
Oil: olive, peanut	1 tsp
Olives	5 small or 2 large
Nuts, other than those listed below	6 small
Almonds	10 whole
Pecans	2 large whole
Peanuts	
Spanish	20 whole
Virginia	10 whole

SATURATED:

Butter	1 tsp
Bacon fat	1 tsp
Bacon, crisp	1 slice
Cream, light	2 tbsp
Cream, heavy whipping	1 tbsp
Cream, sour	2 tbsp
Cream cheese	1 tbsp
Creamer, nondairy	1 tbsp
Margarine, Borden's Danish	1 tsp
Salt pork	3/4″ cube

Appendix B

Some of the multiple vitamin and mineral supplements currently closest to the adult recommendations on page 158 are Insurance Formula (Bronson), Centrum (Lederle), Myadec (Parke-Davis) and One-A-Day Plus Minerals (Miles). Centrum, Myadec, and One-a-Day Plus Minerals are widely available in neighborhood pharmacies. Insurance Formula is available by mail order from Bronson Pharmaceuticals, 4526 Rinetti Lane, La Canada, CA 91011.

There are fewer well-balanced formulas available for children. Insurance Formula (Bronson) can be recommended because both the regular and the chewable tablets come divided into several tabs for the daily dose. This allows you to adjust the amount taken more closely to your needs. Paladec with Minerals (Parke-Davis) is less well balanced, but is the next most complete formulation for children based on these recommendations.

TABLE B-1. Recommended nutritional supplement formulae.

NUTRIENTS	AVERAGE RDA (1–10 yrs)	RECOM. FORMULA (1–10 yrs)	AVERAGE RDA (11+ yrs)	RECOM. FORMULA (11+ yrs)
vitamin A	1780 IU*	1780 IU*	3000 IU*	3000 IU*
vitamin D	400 IU**	200 IU**	300 IU**	150 IU**
vitamin E	9 IU***	9 IU***	15 IU***	15 IU***
thiamine	0.9 mg	0.9 mg	1.2 mg	1.2 mg
riboflavin	1.1 mg	1.1 mg	1.4 mg	1.4 mg
niacin	12.0 mg	12.0 mg	16.0 mg	16.0 mg
vitamin B-6	1.3 mg	1.3 mg	2.0 mg	2.0 mg
vitamin B-12	2.5 mcg	2.5 mcg	3.0 mcg	3.0 mcg
folic acid	200 mcg	200 mcg	400 mcg	400 mcg
biotin	90 mcg	90 mcg	150 mcg	150 mcg
pantothenic acid	3.5 mg	3.5 mg	5.5 mg	5.5 mg
vitamin C	45 mg	90 mg	58 mg	116 mg
calcium	800 mg	240 mg	960 mg	320 mg
magnesium	200 mg	150 mg	330 mg	248 mg
iron	12 mg	12 mg	15 mg	15 mg
zinc	10 mg	10 mg	15 mg	15 mg
iodine	93 mcg	93 mcg	150 mcg	150 mcg
copper	1.8 mg	1.8 mg	2.5 mg	2.5 mg
chromium	83 mcg	83 mcg	125 mcg	125 mcg
selenium	83 mcg	50 mcg	125 mcg	75 mcg

*1 IU vitamin A is equivalent to 0.3 mcg retinol; 3.33 IU vitamin A is equivalent to 1 mcg retinol (as preformed vitamin, does not include carotene)

**400 IU vitamin D is equivalent to 10 mcg cholecalciferol

***1.49 IU vitamin E is equivalent to 1 mg d-alpha-tocopherol

Appendix C: Suggested Reading List

Nutrition Survival Kit
Kathy Dinaburg and D'Ann Akel, Panjandrum, 1976, 248 pages, $5.95; also Jove (Harcourt Brace Jovanovich), 1978, 284 pages, $1.75.

A well-documented and very readable book about nutrition, whole and processed foods, and how they affect your health. Slightly biased toward vegetarianism, this volume offers very practical information plus recipes for people interested in eating more underprocessed foods.

The Supermarket Handbook
Nikki and David Goldbeck, Signet, 1976, 460 pages, $1.95.

Now what do I buy? The answers are all here in this book. Good nutrition is on your market shelves. This guide will help you scout the aisles for nutritious, unprocessed foods. It advises many brand name products and it also supplies some tasty recipes. (Despite this book's recommendation of raw milk, we suggest you continue to use pasteurized milk, to avoid the possibility of contamination.)

The American Way of Life Need Not be Hazardous to Your Health
John Farquhar, M.D., Stanford Alumni Association, P.O. Box 2330, Stanford CA 94305, 1978, 193 pages, $4.95.

This book examines all the risk factors for disease. It includes several chapters on diet and weight control, and also some very useful "game plans" for changing your style of eating. Highly recommended.

Eating Your Way Through Life
Judith Wurtman, Raven Press, 1979, 209 pages, $9.50.

A witty book that explains nutritional needs for people of all ages. It offers a common sense approach to eating and dieting. The book is also a good resource for the consumer, since it deals with such issues as food labeling, popular diets, food advertising, and food fortification and enrichment.

Laurel's Kitchen
Laurel Robertson, Carol Flinders, and Bronwen Godfrey, Nilgiri Press, 1976, 508 pages, $13.95, or paperback by Bantam, 1978, 641 pages, $3.95.

A wonderful book for those interested in learning more about vegetarian diets. Very comprehensive. Includes tasty lowfat recipes and menus. Especially helpful for those wishing to do more baking with whole grains. Also includes food composition tables.

The Anti-Cancer Diet
Donald Germann, Wyden, 1977, 305 pages, $8.95.

A well-referenced and readable review of the current literature on the role of nutrition in the prevention of cancer. The author is a medical doctor (radiologist) who believes strongly in preventive medicine. Recipes are also included.

Permanent Weight Control
Michael and Kathy Mahoney, Norton, 1976, 177 pages, $7.95.

Too often people go on diets, then off diets, and yoyo between weight loss and weight gain. This book deals with weight loss from a behavioral point of view, stressing that food-related behaviors are the key to keeping weight off. ¡This is a down to earth book that will help you "tune in" to your fat behavior patterns. Suggestions for building new eating habits are included. It is not a calorie counter but a consciousness raiser.

Habits Not Diets
James Ferguson, Bull Publishing, 1978, 252 pages, $7.95.

Another book dealing with the behavior patterns of the overweight. It is a do-it-yourself manual for changing your behaviors into ones that promote being thin.

A Change For Heart
James Ferguson and C. Taylor, Bull Publishing, 1978, 183 pages, $4.95.

Gives practical advice on how to change your kitchen into one where healthy foods are stored and prepared. Lists step by step instructions to take the uncertainty out of your efforts to adopt better cooking and eating habits.

Light Style
Rose Dosti, Deborah Kidushim, and Mark Wolke, Harper & Row, 1979, 310 pages, $12.95.

This timely cookbook features lowfat, lowsalt, lowsugar gourmet fare. The recipes appear easy to prepare and wholesome, though we would like to have seen more featuring whole-wheat flour. Calories, sodium, fat, and cholesterol, as well as nutritional exchanges, are noted for each serving.

Diet for a Happy Heart
Jeanne Jones, 101 Productions, 1975, 192 pages, $4.95.

More tasty, lowfat and low cholesterol recipes to add to your collection. Each recipe notes the calories and cholesterol per serving.

The American Heart Association Cookbook
Ballantine, 1979, 403 pages, $2.50.

More recipes, many of your old favorites modified to be lower in saturated fat and cholesterol. Unfortunately, some of the recipes are still high in total fat and sugar.

Cuisine Minceur
Michael Guerrard, Bantam, 1977, 314 pages, $2.50.

For the gourmet cook, some more excellent lowfat recipes with all the subtlety of French cuisine.

Environmental Nutrition
52 Riverside Drive, Suite 15-A, New York, NY 10024, $8.50/6 issues.

A very readable newsletter filled with helpful nutrition information. Written by Registered Dietitians and published bimonthly.

Nutrition Action
Center for Science in the Public Interest (CSPI), 1755 S Street, NW, Washington, DC 20009, $10/12 issues.

Another readable newsletter filled with practical nutrition information. Encourages your involvement in improving the nutrition consciousness of your community, with practical suggestions toward that end.

Bibliography

ALMY, T.P., and D.A. HOWELL, "Diverticular Disease of the Colon," *New England Journal of Medicine*, 302, no. 6 (1980), 324.

AMERICAN DIABETES ASSOCIATION and THE AMERICAN DIETETIC ASSOCIATION, *Exchange Lists for Meal Planning*. New York: American Diabetes Association, 1976.

ANDERSON, J.W., and W.-J.L. CHEN, "Plant Fiber. Carbohydrate and Lipid Metabolism," *American Journal of Clinical Nutrition*, 32 (1979), 346–63.

ANONYMOUS, "Alcohol-Induced Brain Damage and its Reversibility," *Nutrition Reviews*, 38, no. 1 (1980), 11–12.

ARMSTRONG, B.; H. CLARKE; C. MARTIN; W. WARD; N. NORMAN, and J. MASAREI, "Urinary Sodium and Blood Pressure in Vegetarians," *American Journal of Clinical Nutrition*, 32 (1979), 2472–76.

BREWSTER, L., and M.F. JACOBSON, *The Changing American Diet.* Washington, DC: Center for Science in the Public Interest, 1978.

BRIGGS, G.M., and D.H. CALLOWAY, "Carbohydrates and Alcohol," *Bogert's Nutrition and Physical Fitness* (10th ed.), pp. 61–62, eds. G.M. Briggs and D.H. Calloway. Philadelphia: Saunders, 1979.

BUNKER, M.L., and M. MCWILLIAMS, "Caffeine Content of Common Beverages," *Journal of the American Dietetic Association,* 74 (1979), 28–31.

BURKITT, D.P.; A.R.P. WALKER, and N.S. PAINTER, "Dietary Fiber and Disease," *Journal of the American Medical Association,* 229 (1974), 1068–74.

CARROLL, K.K., "Experimental Evidence of Dietary Factors and Hormone-Dependent Cancers," *Cancer Research,* 35 (1975), 3374–83.

COHEN, S., and G.H. BOOTH, "Gastric Acid Secretion and Lower-Esophageal-Sphincter Pressure in Response to Coffee and Caffeine," *New England Journal of Medicine,* 293 (1975), 897.

CROSBY, W.H., "Lead-Contaminated Health Food," *Journal of the American Medical Association,* 237 (1977), 2627–29.

EMKEN, E.A., and H.J. DUTTON (eds.), *Geometrical and Positional Fatty Acid Isomers.* Champaign, Ill: American Oil Chemists Society, 1979.

FOOD and NUTRITION BOARD NATIONAL RESEARCH COUNCIL, *Recommended Dietary Allowances.* Washington, DC: National Academy of Sciences, 1980.

GEAR, J.S.S.; P. FURSDON; D.J. NOLAN; A. WARE; J.I. MANN; A.J.M. BRODRIBB, and M.P. VESSEY, "Symptomless Diverticular Disease and Intake of Dietary Fiber," *Lancet,* 2 (1979), 511–14.

GORI, G.B., "Dietary and Nutritional Implications in the Multi-factorial Etiology of Certain Prevalent Human Cancers," *Cancer,* 43 (May 1979 supplement), 2151–61.

GRANDE, F., "Sugars in Cardiovascular Disease," *Sugars in Nutrition,* pp. 401-437, eds. H.L. Sipple and K.W. McNutt. New York: Academic Press, 1974.

HATHCOCK, J.N., and J. COON (eds.), *Nutrition and Drug Interrelationships.* New York: Academic Press, 1978.

KAY, R.M., "Food Form, Postprandial Glycemia, and Satiety," *American Journal of Clinical Nutrition,* 31 (1978), 738–41.

KELSAY, J.L.; K.M. BEHALL, and E.S. PRATHER, "Effect of Fiber from Fruits and Vegetables on Metabolic Responses of Human Subjects. 1. Bowel

Transit Times, Number of Defecations, Fecal Weight, Urinary Excretions of Energy and Nitrogen and Apparent Digestibilities of Energy, Nitrogen and Fat," *American Journal of Clinical Nutrition*, 31 (1978), 1149–53.

LAPORTE, R.E.; J.L. CRESANTA, and L.H. KULLER, "The Relationship of Alcohol Consumption to Atherosclerotic Heart Disease," *Preventive Medicine*, 9 (1980), 22–40.

MARSH, A.G.; T.V. SANCHEZ; O. MICKELSEN; J. KEISER, and G. MAYOR, "Cortical Bone Density of Adult Lacto-Ovo-Vegetarian and Omnivorous Women," *Journal of the American Dietetic Association*, 76 (1980), 148–51.

MENDELSON, J. H., and N. MELLO, "Biologic Concomitants of Alcoholism," *New England Journal of Medicine*, 301, no. 17 (1979), 912–21.

MENEELEY, G.R., and H.D. BATTARBEE, "Sodium and Potassium," *Nutrition Reviews*, 34, no. 8 (1976), 225–35.

MILLER, A.B., "Nutrition and Cancer," *Preventive Medicine*, 9 (1980), 189–96.

MINTON, J.P.; M.K. FOECKING; D.J.T. WEBSTER, and R.H. MATTHEWS, "Caffeine, Cyclic Nucleotides, and Breast Disease," *Surgery*, 86, no. 1 (1979), 105–09.

PAGE, L., and B. FRIEND, "The Changing American Diet," *Bioscience*, 28, no. 3 (1978), 192–97.

PHILLIPS, R.L., "Role of Lifestyle and Dietary Habits in Risk of Cancer Among Seventh-Day Adventists," *Cancer Research*, 35 (1975), 3513–22.

PHILLIPS, R.L.; F.R. LEMON; W.L. BEESON, and J.W. KUZMA, "Coronary Heart Disease Mortality Among Seventh-Day Adventists with Differing Dietary Habits: A Preliminary Report," *American Journal of Clinical Nutrition*, 31 (October 1978 supplement), 191–98.

ROBERTSON, D.; J.C. FROLICH; R.K. CARR; J.T. WATSON; J.W. HOLLIFIELD, et al., "Effects of Caffeine on Plasma Renin Activity, Catecholamines and Blood Pressure," *New England Journal of Medicine*, 298, no. 4 (1978), 181–86.

SACKS, F.M., B. ROSNER, and E.H. KASS, "Blood Pressure in Vegetarians," *American Journal of Epidemiology*, 100 (1974), 390–98.

SACKS, F.M.; W.P. CASTELLI; A. DONNER, and E.H. KASS, "Plasma Lipids and Lipoproteins in Vegetarians and Controls," *New England Journal of Medicine*, 292 (1975), 1148–51.

SENATE COMMITTEE ON NUTRITION AND HUMAN NEEDS, UNITED STATES SENATE, *Dietary Goals for the United States*, 2nd ed. Washington, DC: Government Printing Office (Stock No. 052-070-04376-8), December 1977.

SHANNON, I.L., "Sugar and Glucose in Dry Breakfast Cereals," *Journal of Dentistry for Children*, September–October 1974.

SHAW, S., and C.S. LIEBER, "Nutrition and Alcoholism," in *Modern Nutrition in Health and Disease*, 6th ed., pp. 1220–43, eds. F.S. Goodhart and M.E. Shils, Philadelphia: Lea & Febiger, 1980.

STEPHENSON, P.E., "Physiologic and Psychotropic Effects of Caffeine on Man," *Journal of the American Dietetic Association*, 71 (1977), 240–47.

STONE, O.J., "Alcoholic Malnutrition and Skin Infections," *Nutrition Today*, November–December, (1978), 6–10, 27–30.

UNITED STATES DEPARTMENT OF AGRICULTURE, UNITED STATES DEPARTMENT OF HEALTH, EDUCATION AND WELFARE, *Nutrition and Your Health—Dietary Guidelines for Americans*. Washington, DC: Government Printing Office, 1980.

Index